# Attention-Deficit/Hyperactivity Disorder in Adults

## About the Authors

**Brian P. Daly**, PhD, is associate professor and department head of psychological and brain sciences at Drexel University. Dr. Daly is past president of the Philadelphia Behavior Therapy Association and recipient of grant funding from the Pew Charitable Trusts, W. K. Kellogg Foundation, Sixers Youth Foundation, Shire Pharmaceuticals, and Justice Resource Institute. He currently serves on the editorial board of Professional Psychology: Research and Practice, as well as on the advisory committees for several nonprofit organizations.

**Michael J. Silverstein**, MS, is a postdoctoral fellow at the Center for Cognitive Behavioral Therapy in Media, PA. His research interests include etiology of trauma symptoms after exposure to acute, chronic, and systemic stressors and the relationship between attention-deficit/hyperactivity disorder and posttraumatic stress disorder in youth. Clinically, Mr. Silverstein is interested in providing empirically based interventions to toddlers, children, adolescents, and their families.

**Ronald T. Brown**, PhD, ABPP, is the Dean of the School of Integrated Health Sciences at the University of Nevada, Las Vegas. Dr. Brown has been the past president of the University of North Texas at Dallas and also is the past president of the Association of Psychologists in Academic Health Centers and the Society of Pediatric Psychology of the American Psychological Association. Dr. Bown has published over 300 articles and chapters as well as 12 books related to childhood psychopathology and pediatric psychology.

## Advances in Psychotherapy – Evidence-Based Practice

### Series Editor
**Danny Wedding**, PhD, MPH, Professor Emeritus, University of Missouri–Saint Louis, MO

### Associate Editors
**Jonathan S. Comer**, PhD, Professor of Psychology and Psychiatry, Director of Mental Health Interventions and Technology (MINT) Program, Center for Children and Families, Florida International University, Miami, FL

**J. Kim Penberthy**, PhD, ABPP, Professor of Psychiatry & Neurobehavioral Sciences, University of Virginia, Charlottesville, VA

**Kenneth E. Freedland**, PhD, Professor of Psychiatry and Psychology, Washington University School of Medicine, St. Louis, MO

**Linda C. Sobell**, PhD, ABPP, Professor, Center for Psychological Studies, Nova Southeastern University, Ft. Lauderdale, FL

The basic objective of this series is to provide therapists with practical, evidence-based treatment guidance for the most common disorders seen in clinical practice – and to do so in a reader-friendly manner. Each book in the series is both a compact "how-to" reference on a particular disorder for use by professional clinicians in their daily work and an ideal educational resource for students as well as for practice-oriented continuing education.

The most important feature of the books is that they are practical and easy to use: All are structured similarly and all provide a compact and easy-to-follow guide to all aspects that are relevant in real-life practice. Tables, boxed clinical "pearls," marginal notes, and summary boxes assist orientation, while checklists provide tools for use in daily practice.

## Continuing Education Credits

Psychologists and other healthcare providers may earn five continuing education credits for reading the books in the *Advances in Psychotherapy* series and taking a multiple-choice exam. This continuing education program is a partnership of Hogrefe Publishing and the National Register of Health Service Psychologists. Details are available at https://www.hogrefe.com/us/cenatreg

The National Register of Health Service Psychologists is approved by the American Psychological Association to sponsor continuing education for psychologists. The National Register maintains responsibility for this program and its content.

Advances in Psychotherapy – Evidence-Based Practice, Volume 35

# Attention-Deficit/ Hyperactivity Disorder in Adults

## 2nd edition

**Brian P. Daly**
Department of Psychological and Brain Sciences, Drexel University, Philadelphia, PA

**Michael J. Silverstein**
Center for Cognitive Behavioral Therapy, Media, PA

**Ronald T. Brown**
School of Integrated Health Sciences, University of Nevada, Las Vegas, NV

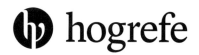

**Library of Congress of Congress Cataloging in Publication** information for the print version of this book is available via the Library of Congress Marc Database under the Library of Congress Control Number 2023951194

**Library and Archives Canada Cataloguing in Publication**

Title: Attention-deficit/hyperactivity disorder in adults / Brian P. Daly, Department of Psychological and Brain Sciences, Drexel University, Philadelphia, PA, Michael J. Silverstein, Center for Cognitive Behavioral Therapy, Media, PA, Ronald T. Brown, School of Integrated Health Sciences, University of Nevada, Las Vegas, NV.

Names: Daly, Brian P., author. | Silverstein, Michael J. (Of the Center for Cognitive Behavioral Therapy in Media), author. | Brown, Ronald T., author.

Series: Advances in psychotherapy--evidence-based practice ; v. 35.

Description: 2nd edition. | Series statement: Advances in psychotherapy--evidence-based practice ; volume 35. | Includes bibliographical references.

Identifiers: Canadiana (print) 20230586627 | Canadiana (ebook) 20230586686 | ISBN 9780889375994 (softcover) | ISBN 9781613345993 (EPUB) | ISBN 9781616765996 (PDF)

Subjects: LCSH: Attention-deficit disorder in adults—Handbooks, manuals, etc. | LCGFT: Handbooks and manuals.

Classification: LCC RC394.A85 D35 2024 | DDC 616.85/89—dc23

© 2024 by Hogrefe Publishing
www.hogrefe.com

The authors and publisher have made every effort to ensure that the information contained in this text is in accord with the current state of scientific knowledge, recommendations, and practice at the time of publication. In spite of this diligence, errors cannot be completely excluded. Also, due to changing regulations and continuing research, information may become outdated at any point. The authors and publisher disclaim any responsibility for any consequences which may follow from the use of information presented in this book.

Registered trademarks are not noted specifically as such in this publication. The use of descriptive names, registered names, and trademarks does not imply, even in the absence of a specific statement, that such names are exempt from the relevant protective laws and regulations and therefore free for general use.

The cover image is an agency photo depicting models. Use of the photo on this publication does not imply any connection between the content of this publication and any person depicted in the cover image.
Cover image: © skynesher – iStock.com

PUBLISHING OFFICES

| | |
|---|---|
| USA: | Hogrefe Publishing Corporation, 44 Merrimac St., Suite 207, Newburyport, MA 01950<br>Phone 978 255 3700; E-mail customersupport@hogrefe.com |
| EUROPE: | Hogrefe Publishing GmbH, Merkelstr. 3, 37085 Göttingen, Germany<br>Phone +49 551 99950 0, Fax +49 551 99950 111; E-mail publishing@hogrefe.com |

SALES & DISTRIBUTION

| | |
|---|---|
| USA: | Hogrefe Publishing, Customer Services Department,<br>30 Amberwood Parkway, Ashland, OH 44805<br>Phone 800 228 3749, Fax 419 281 6883; E-mail customersupport@hogrefe.com |
| UK: | Hogrefe Publishing, c/o Marston Book Services Ltd., 160 Eastern Ave.,<br>Milton Park, Abingdon, OX14 4SB<br>Phone +44 1235 465577, Fax +44 1235 465556; E-mail direct.orders@marston.co.uk |
| EUROPE: | Hogrefe Publishing, Merkelstr. 3, 37085 Göttingen, Germany<br>Phone +49 551 99950 0, Fax +49 551 99950 111; E-mail publishing@hogrefe.com |

OTHER OFFICES

| | |
|---|---|
| CANADA: | Hogrefe Publishing Corporation, 82 Laird Drive, East York, Ontario, M4G 3V1 |
| SWITZERLAND: | Hogrefe Publishing, Länggass-Strasse 76, 3012 Bern |

No part of this book may be reproduced, stored in a retrieval system or transmitted, in any form or by any means, electronic, mechanical, photocopying, microfilming, recording or otherwise, without written permission from the publisher.

Printed and bound in the USA

ISBN 978-0-88937-599-4 (print) · ISBN 978-1-61676-599-6 (PDF) · ISBN 978-1-61334-599-3 (EPUB)
https://doi.org/10.1027/00599-000

# Acknowledgments

Brian P. Daly is grateful for the love, grace, and laughter from Tina, Leo, Sofie-Mathilde, and Colt. Having the puzzle pieces fit so snuggly together makes me happy every day.

Michael J. Silverstein wishes to thank his wife Gila, parents Aliza and Len, and mentor Dr. Daly for their support and guidance.

Ronald T. Brown recognizes the extraordinary mentorship of Lorene C. Pilcher who began to ignite the flame of a love for scholarship and the study of individuals with attention-deficit/hyperactivity disorder.

# Contents

Acknowledgments .................................................... v

| | | |
|---|---|---|
| **1** | **Description** ............................................ | 1 |
| 1.1 | Terminology ............................................. | 1 |
| 1.2 | Definition ............................................... | 2 |
| 1.2.1 | Diagnostic Criteria ..................................... | 2 |
| 1.2.2 | Applicability of Criteria for Adults ..................... | 5 |
| 1.3 | Epidemiology ........................................... | 5 |
| 1.3.1 | Prevalence and Incidence ............................... | 5 |
| 1.3.2 | Sex ..................................................... | 6 |
| 1.3.3 | Age ..................................................... | 6 |
| 1.3.4 | Ethnicity ................................................ | 6 |
| 1.4 | Course and Prognosis ................................... | 7 |
| 1.5 | Differential Diagnosis ................................... | 8 |
| 1.5.1 | Disruptive, Impulse-Control, and Conduct Disorders ..... | 8 |
| 1.5.2 | Depressive Disorders .................................... | 9 |
| 1.5.3 | Anxiety Disorders ....................................... | 10 |
| 1.5.4 | Trauma- and Stress-Related Disorders ................... | 10 |
| 1.5.5 | Bipolar and Related Disorders ........................... | 10 |
| 1.5.6 | Personality Disorders ................................... | 11 |
| 1.5.7 | Substance-Related and Addictive Disorders .............. | 11 |
| 1.5.8 | Neurodevelopmental, Physical, and Medical Conditions .. | 12 |
| 1.5.9 | Environmental and Psychosocial Factors ................. | 13 |
| 1.6 | Comorbidity ............................................. | 14 |
| 1.6.1 | Oppositional Defiant and Conduct Disorders ............. | 15 |
| 1.6.2 | Depressive Disorders .................................... | 16 |
| 1.6.3 | Anxiety Disorders ....................................... | 17 |
| 1.6.4 | Learning Disabilities .................................... | 17 |
| 1.6.5 | Bipolar and Related Disorders ........................... | 18 |
| 1.6.6 | Substance-Related and Addictive Disorders .............. | 19 |
| 1.6.7 | Personality Disorders ................................... | 19 |
| 1.6.8 | Sleep–Wake Disorders ................................... | 20 |
| 1.7 | Diagnostic Procedures and Documentation ............... | 21 |
| 1.7.1 | Diagnostic Interviews ................................... | 22 |
| 1.7.2 | Rating Scales ............................................ | 23 |
| 1.7.3 | Psychoeducational Testing ............................... | 25 |
| 1.7.4 | Neuropsychological Testing .............................. | 25 |
| 1.7.5 | Laboratory Testing ...................................... | 26 |

| 2 | **Theories and Models of ADHD in Adults** | 27 |
|---|---|---|
| 2.1 | Neurobiological Factors in ADHD | 27 |
| 2.1.1 | Genetic Contributions | 27 |
| 2.1.2 | Neurological Factors | 28 |
| 2.1.3 | Cognitive Determinants | 30 |
| 2.2 | Environmental Risk Factors | 30 |
| 2.2.1 | Biological Adversity Factors | 31 |
| 2.2.2 | Environmental Toxins | 32 |
| 2.2.3 | Food Additives/Dietary Factors | 32 |
| 2.3 | Psychosocial Adversity Factors | 32 |
| 2.4 | Interactions Between Neurobiological, Environmental, and Psychosocial Adversity Factors | 33 |
| 3 | **Diagnosis and Treatment Indications** | 35 |
| 3.1 | Assessment Procedures | 36 |
| 3.1.1 | General Considerations | 36 |
| 3.1.2 | Developmental History | 37 |
| 3.1.3 | Clinical Interview | 38 |
| 3.1.4 | Behavioral Rating Scales | 40 |
| 3.1.5 | Differential Diagnosis/Comorbidities | 41 |
| 3.1.6 | Testing | 42 |
| 3.2 | The Decision-Making Process | 43 |
| 3.3 | Treatment Considerations | 45 |
| 4 | **Treatment** | 47 |
| 4.1 | Methods of Treatment | 47 |
| 4.1.1 | Psychopharmacology | 48 |
| 4.1.2 | Stimulant Medications | 50 |
| 4.1.3 | Nonstimulant Medications | 53 |
| 4.1.4 | Psychosocial and Psychological Therapies | 55 |
| 4.1.5 | Coaching and CBT | 55 |
| 4.1.6 | Metacognitive Therapy: Time-Management and Organizational-Skills Training | 56 |
| 4.1.7 | Supportive and Family Therapies | 57 |
| 4.1.8 | Neurofeedback and Cognitive-Enhancement Training | 57 |
| 4.1.9 | Psychoeducation | 58 |
| 4.2 | Mechanisms of Action | 58 |
| 4.3 | Efficacy and Prognosis | 60 |
| 4.4 | Variations and Combinations of Methods | 63 |
| 4.5 | Problems in Carrying Out the Treatments | 66 |
| 4.6 | Multicultural Issues | 67 |
| 5 | **Case Vignettes** | 69 |
| 6 | **Further Reading** | 73 |
| 7 | **References** | 74 |
| 8 | **Appendix: Tools and Resources** | 89 |

# 1

# Description

## 1.1 Terminology

Attention-deficit/hyperactivity disorder (ADHD) is a neurodevelopmental disorder marked by persistent patterns of inattention and/or hyperactivity-impulsivity symptoms that emerge during childhood and are functionally impairing across settings. This book recognizes that the disorder can persist over the life span and well into adulthood. The *Diagnostic and Statistical Manual of Mental Disorders* (5th ed.; *DSM-5*; American Psychiatric Association [APA], 2013) assigns the following codes for this disorder:
- 314.01 Attention-Deficit/Hyperactivity Disorder, Combined Presentation
- 314.00 Attention-Deficit/Hyperactivity Disorder, Predominantly Inattentive Presentation
- 314.01 Attention-Deficit/Hyperactivity Disorder, Predominantly Hyperactive/Impulsive Presentation
- 314.01 Other Specified Attention-Deficit/Hyperactivity Disorder
- 314.01 Unspecified Attention-Deficit/Hyperactivity Disorder

The *International Classification of Diseases* (10th rev., clinical modification; *ICD-10-CM*; World Health Organization, 2021) lists ADHD under the following codes:
- F90.0 Attention-Deficit/Hyperactivity Disorder, Predominantly Inattentive Type
- F90.1 Attention-Deficit/Hyperactivity Disorder, Predominantly Hyperactive Type
- F90.2 Attention-Deficit/Hyperactivity Disorder, Combined Type
- F90.8 Attention-Deficit/Hyperactivity Disorder, Other Type
- F90.9 Attention-Deficit/Hyperactivity Disorder, Unspecified Type

First described within the medical literature in the late 1700s (Barkley & Peters, 2012), ADHD-related symptoms were previously referred to by labels including "minimal brain damage," "minimal brain dysfunction," "hyperkinetic impulse disorder," "hyperactive child syndrome," "hyperkinetic reaction of childhood," and "attention deficit disorder," among others (Taylor, 2011). Changes in terminology generally reflect evolving theoretical conceptions based on etiology, symptoms of the disorder, and its management.

## 1.2 Definition

### 1.2.1 Diagnostic Criteria

According to the *DSM-5* (American Psychiatric Association, 2022), ADHD represents "a persistent pattern of inattention and/or hyperactivity-impulsivity that interferes with functioning or development" as defined by the following diagnostic criteria:

---

**Box 1**
**DSM-5-TR Diagnostic Criteria for ADHD**

**A.** Either 1 and/or 2:
1. **Inattention:** Six (or more) of the following symptoms have persisted for at least 6 months to a degree that is inconsistent with developmental level and that negatively impacts directly on social and academic/occupational activities. *Note:* The symptoms are not solely a manifestation of oppositional behavior, defiance, hostility, or failure to understand tasks or instructions. For older adolescents and adults (ages 17 and older), at least five symptoms are required.
   a. Often fails to give close attention to details or makes careless mistakes in schoolwork, at work, or during other activities (e.g., overlooks or misses details, work is inaccurate).
   b. Often has difficulty sustaining attention in tasks or play activities (e.g., has difficulty remaining focused during lectures, conversations, or lengthy reading).
   c. Often does not seem to listen when spoken to directly (e.g., mind seems elsewhere, even in the absence of any obvious distraction).
   d. Often does not follow through on instructions and fails to finish schoolwork, chores, or duties in the workplace (e.g., starts tasks but quickly loses focus and is easily distracted or sidetracked).
   e. Often has difficulty organizing tasks and activities (e.g., difficulty managing sequential tasks; difficulty keeping materials and belongings in order; messy, disorganized work; has poor time management; fails to meet deadlines).
   f. Often avoids, dislikes, or is reluctant to engage in tasks that require sustained mental effort (e.g., schoolwork or homework; for older adolescents and adults, preparing reports, completing forms, reviewing lengthy papers).
   g. Often loses things necessary for tasks or activities (e.g., school materials, pencils, books, tools, wallets, keys, paperwork, eyeglasses, cell phones).
   h. Is often easily distracted by extraneous stimuli (for older adolescents and adults, may include unrelated thoughts).
   i. Is often forgetful in daily activities (e.g., doing chores, running errands; for older adolescents and adults, returning calls, paying bills, keeping appointments).
2. **Hyperactivity and impulsivity:** Six (or more) of the following symptoms have persisted for at least 6 months to a degree that is inconsistent with developmental level and that negatively impacts directly on social and academic/occupational activities. *Note:* The symptoms are not solely a manifestation of oppositional behavior, defiance, hostility, or a failure to understand tasks or instructions. For older adolescents and adults (ages 17 and older), at least five symptoms are required.

a. Often fidgets with or taps hands or feet or squirms in seat.
   b. Often leaves seat in situations when remaining seated is expected (e.g., leaves his or her place in the classroom, in the office or other workplace, or in other situations that require remaining in place).
   c. Often runs about or climbs in situations where it is inappropriate. (*Note:* In adolescents or adults, may be limited to feeling restless).
   d. Often unable to play or engage in leisure activities quietly.
   e. Is often "on the go," acting as if "driven by a motor" (e.g., is unable to be or uncomfortable being still for extended time, as in restaurants, meetings; may be experienced by others as being restless or difficult to keep up with).
   f. Often talks excessively.
   g. Often blurts out an answer before a question has been completed (e.g., completes people's sentences, cannot wait for his or her turn in conversations).
   h. Often has difficulty waiting his or her turn (e.g., while waiting in line).
   i. Often interrupts or intrudes on others (e.g., butts into conversations, games, or activities; may start using other people's things without asking or receiving permission; for adolescents and adults, may intrude into or take over what others are doing

**B.** Several inattentive or hyperactive-impulsive symptoms were present prior to age 12 years.

**C.** Several inattentive or hyperactive-impulsive symptoms are present in two or more settings (e.g., at home, school, or work; with friends or relatives; in other activities).

**D.** There is clear evidence that the symptoms interfere with, or reduce the quality of, social, academic, or occupational functioning.

**E.** The symptoms do not occur exclusively during the course of schizophrenia or another psychotic disorder and are not better explained by another mental disorder (e.g., mood disorder, anxiety disorder, dissociative disorder, personality disorder, substance intoxication or withdrawal).

*Specify whether:*

**314.01(F90.2) Combined presentation:** If both Criterion A1 (inattention) and Criterion A2 (hyperactivity-impulsivity) are met for the past 6 months.

**314.00(F90.0) Predominantly inattentive presentation:** If Criterion A1 (inattention) is met but Criterion A2 (hyperactivity-impulsivity) is not met for the past 6 months.

**314.01(F90.1) Predominantly hyperactive/impulsive presentation:** If Criterion A2 (hyperactivity-impulsivity) is met and Criterion A1 (inattention) is not met for the past 6 months.

*Specify whether:*

**314.01(F90.2) Combined presentation:** If both Criterion A1 (inattention) and Criterion A2 (hyperactivity-impulsivity) are met for the past 6 months.

**314.00(F90.0) Predominantly inattentive presentation:** If Criterion A1 (inattention) is met but Criterion A2 (hyperactivity-impulsivity) is not met for the past 6 months.

**314.01(F90.1) Predominantly hyperactive/impulsive presentation:** If Criterion A2 (hyperactivity-impulsivity) is met and Criterion A1 (inattention) is not met for the past 6 months.

*Specify if:*

**In partial remission:** When full criteria were previously met, fewer than the full criteria have been met for the past 6 months, and the symptoms still result in impairment in social, academic, or occupational functioning.

*Specify current severity:*

**Mild:** Few, if any, symptoms in excess of those required to make the diagnosis are present, and symptoms result in no more than minor impairments in social or occupational functioning.

**Moderate:** Symptoms or functional impairment between "mild" and "severe" are present.

**Severe:** Many symptoms in excess of those required to make the diagnosis, or several symptoms that are particularly severe, are present, or the symptoms result in marked impairment in social or occupational functioning.

Reprinted with permission from the *Diagnostic and Statistical Manual of Mental Disorders* (5th ed., text. rev.), https://doi.org/10.1176/appi.books.9780890425787 (Copyright © 2022). American Psychiatric Association. All Rights Reserved.

According to *ICD-10-CM* (World Health Organization, 2019), the diagnostic criteria for ADHD are specified in Box 2.

### Box 2
### ICD-10-CM Diagnostic Criteria for ADHD

**F90. Hyperkinetic Disorders:** A group of disorders characterized by an early onset (usually in the first five years of life), lack of persistence in activities that require cognitive involvement, and a tendency to move from one activity to another without completing any one, together with disorganized, ill-regulated, and excessive activity. Several other abnormalities may be associated. Hyperkinetic children are often reckless and impulsive, prone to accidents, and find themselves in disciplinary trouble because of unthinking breaches of rules rather than deliberate defiance. Their relationships with adults are often socially disinhibited, with a lack of normal caution and reserve. They are unpopular with other children and may become isolated. Impairment of cognitive functions is common, and specific delays in motor and language development are disproportionately frequent. Secondary complications include dissocial behavior and low self-esteem.

*Excludes:*
  Anxiety disorders
  Mood [affective] disorders
  Pervasive developmental disorders
  Schizophrenia

**F90.0 Disturbance of activity and attention:**

Attention deficit:
  Disorder with hyperactivity
  Hyperactivity disorder
  Syndrome with hyperactivity

*Excludes:*
  Hyperkinetic disorder associated with conduct disorder

Reprinted with permission from the *ICD-10-CM Classification of Mental and Behavioral Disorders*, https://icd.who.int/browse10/2019/en#/F90 (Copyright © 2019). World Health Organization. All Rights Reserved.

### 1.2.2 Applicability of Criteria for Adults

It is important to note that ADHD criteria in previous editions of the *DSM* and *ICD* were initially designed for children, and controversy exists regarding the appropriateness of the nomenclature for adults (Kessler et al., 2010). Most prominently, the diagnostic requirement of childhood onset of symptoms in the *DSM-5* (i.e., some symptoms present before the age of 12 years) and *ICD-10* (i.e., symptoms usually in the first 5 years of life) can be very difficult for a clinician to assess retrospectively when conducting a diagnostic assessment with an adult (Sharma et al., 2021). In addition, the presentation of ADHD symptoms may differ considerably between adults and children (Vitola et al., 2017). For instance, ADHD among adults appears to be better characterized by deficits in executive functioning and attention relative to hyperactivity or impulsivity that is more frequently present among children and adolescents. Moreover, some research suggests fewer symptoms are needed to reliably identify adults with ADHD (Kessler et al., 2010; Vitola et al., 2017). Considering these concerns, the *DSM* committee reduced the symptom threshold from six in the *Diagnostic and Statistical Manual of Mental Disorders Text Revision* (4th ed.; *DSM-IV-TR*; APA, 2000) to five in the *DSM-5* for adults over the age of 17 years (APA, 2013), a change that persists in the *Diagnostic and Statistical Manual of Mental Disorders Text Revision* (5th ed.; *DSM-5-TR*; APA, 2022). Despite the importance of executive function among adults with ADHD (Adler et al., 2015; Silverstein et al., 2020), the ADHD symptom list itself was not expanded in *DSM-5* or *DSM-5-TR* to include more features of executive dysfunction.

## 1.3 Epidemiology

### 1.3.1 Prevalence and Incidence

Although ADHD was once believed to primarily be a childhood condition, the disorder is now increasingly recognized as one of the most common mental health conditions in adults. Depending on the population, reports indicate prevalence rates between 2% and 5% (Asherson et al., 2016). Notably, there are some data to suggest increasing rates of ADHD diagnosis among adults in the US (Chung et al., 2019). For example, findings from a recent cohort study by Chung and colleagues (2019) indicated the annual adult ADHD prevalence and incidence rates had increased over a 10-year period from 0.43% in 2007 to 0.96% in 2016. Findings from a 2017 global sample that looked at the aggregate prevalence of ADHD in adults in 20 countries revealed a prevalence rate of 2.8% (Fayyad et al., 2017). A consistent finding across studies from the US and global populations was higher prevalence rates among adults living in higher-income countries (Chung et al., 2019; Fayyad et al., 2017).

### 1.3.2 Sex

ADHD is diagnosed more frequently in adult males than in females (Chung et al., 2019), but these sex differences are less prominent in adults as compared to children (Simon et al., 2009). Several proposed explanations for the narrowing in sex ratio between child- and adult-diagnosed ADHD include higher disease persistence among females (Hinshaw et al., 2012) as compared to males (Biederman et al., 2012), difference in the symptom presentation of males (e.g., more likely to present with combined symptoms and higher rates of hyperactivity and impulsivity) as compared to females (e.g., more likely to present with inattentive symptoms; Li et al., 2019), and different patterns of comorbidity (e.g., males more likely to present with externalizing disorders and females more likely to present with internalizing disorders; Williamson & Johnston, 2015).

### 1.3.3 Age

ADHD is typically first identified during the preschool or elementary years, when functionally impairing symptoms become evident to parents and teachers (APA, 2013; Kooij et al., 2010). Many adults who were diagnosed with ADHD as children report their symptoms have diminished with age; however, it is estimated that 35–65% of adults diagnosed with ADHD during childhood will continue to meet full criteria for the disorder (Owens et al., 2015). Although ADHD research has historically focused on adults who were first diagnosed as children, a growing number of adults are seeking initial evaluation and treatment for inattention (Huang et al., 2020). Some experts maintain that the disorder remains underrecognized in adults secondary to more subtle symptom presentations, stigma, and the frequency of comorbid psychiatric conditions (Ginsberg et al., 2014).

### 1.3.4 Ethnicity

*ADHD occurs across all nationalities and cultures*

ADHD has been reported in adults across cultures and nationalities. For example, the World Health Organization World Mental Health Surveys that screened for ADHD in selected countries in the Americas, Europe, and the Middle East found prevalence rates of 0.6% (Iraq and Romania) to 7.3% (France) (Fayyad et al., 2017). As mentioned previously, higher prevalence rates were identified in higher-income countries such as France and the Netherlands (Fayyad et al., 2017). More recent studies have examined relationships between race, ethnicity, and adult ADHD within the US. Findings from Chung and colleagues (2019) suggested that within the US, ADHD is more prevalent among White populations as compared to non-Hispanic Black or Hispanic/Latino populations with Asian and Native Hawaiian or other Pacific Islander adults having the lowest rates.

## 1.4 Course and Prognosis

ADHD is considered a chronic disorder in which symptoms present before the age of 12 years (APA, 2022). Approximately 60% of adults diagnosed with ADHD during childhood continue to experience some level of clinically significant symptom impairment through adulthood (Targum & Adler, 2014). Notably, the extant literature suggests that symptom presentation has a distinct course as individuals age. In adulthood, hyperactivity tends to decrease in severity as inattention, restlessness, and impulsivity become more prominent with age (Targum & Adler, 2014). In fact, of those adults diagnosed with ADHD during childhood, the majority (90%) experience inattention, whereas only half (50%) report problems with hyperactivity and/or impulsivity. More persistent symptoms are associated with higher familial rates of ADHD (for a review, see Faraone & Larsson, 2019).

Without appropriate symptom management, ADHD during adulthood can negatively impact academic, social, and work functioning (Holst & Thorell, 2019). For example, adult ADHD each year results in incremental costs that range from $105 to $194 billion (Doshi et al., 2012), and adults with ADHD also report significantly lower academic achievement and educational attainment (Arnold et al., 2020) relative to their typically developing peers. These individuals may present in school and work settings as distractible, disorganized, and sensitive to stress, all factors that can compromise advancement and achievement (Kooij et al., 2010). Another factor closely related to the prognosis of ADHD in adulthood is the prevalence of comorbid mental health disorders with findings suggesting that as many as 50-80% of adults with ADHD have, or will develop, at least one coexisting psychiatric disorder (Katzman et al., 2017). An estimated 57% of adults with ADHD meet criteria for a depressive disorder, 66% meet criteria for an anxiety disorder, and 9% have comorbid alcohol use disorder while 16% have a drug use disorder (Chung et al., 2019). Prognosis may also be impacted by family functioning in childhood, in terms of the environmental impact on development of comorbid conduct issues and other mental health concerns (APA, 2022).

Relatively poor outcomes reported for adults with ADHD must be interpreted considering experts' suspicions that underrecognition of the disorder has led to underdiagnosis and inadequate treatment (Ginsberg et al., 2014). Indeed, Kessler and colleagues (2006) reported that of 3,199 American adults with ADHD, only 10.9% had received treatment for ADHD within the previous year. However, outcomes in adults with ADHD who receive appropriate treatment (to be discussed in later chapters of this volume) are encouraging. For example, psychosocial and pharmacological interventions for adult ADHD can produce improvements in quality of life and symptom reductions (McGough, 2016). Unfortunately, these interventions are not curative: Effective management of adult ADHD is likely to require long-term psychological and psychopharmacological management (McGough, 2016).

## 1.5 Differential Diagnosis

Differential diagnosis in adults with ADHD is a formidable task for even the most seasoned practitioners because of the comorbidities frequently found among adults with the disorder (Evans et al., 2021). It has been our clinical experience that many adults suspect that they have ADHD when their children are initially identified with the disorder or when they are seeking expert mental health care for psychiatric problems associated with depression, anxiety, or addiction problems. The precise diagnosis of ADHD is made exceedingly complicated by the fact that numerous neuropsychiatric, substance abuse, medical, and physical disorders frequently share similar symptoms to ADHD and, thus, the skilled practitioner needs to distinguish these anxiety-related symptoms from the traditional symptoms associated with ADHD (see Section 1.2.1). Those categories in which there may be frequent symptomatic overlap include mood disorders (e.g., anxiety, depression, posttraumatic stress disorder [PTSD], bipolar disorder), personality disorders (e.g., borderline and antisocial personality disorder), substance abuse disorders (e.g., alcohol, cocaine, and other drug abuse), neurological disorders (seizure disorders), physical or medical conditions (e.g., acquired traumatic brain injury, endocrine and metabolic disorders, sleep apnea), and, finally, psychosocial and environmental factors that may be associated with several ADHD symptoms (e.g., trauma, stress, sudden life change, grief). Because the symptoms associated with these aforementioned conditions may mirror symptoms related to ADHD, the astute practitioner must consider alternative explanations, and when appropriate must diagnose each condition separately because each diagnosis may require a unique modality of management and treatment. Simultaneously, the practitioner must continue to rule out any somatic symptoms that may in fact mimic symptoms associated with ADHD.

It also must be noted that the natural history of ADHD suggests that it is a long course disorder where there is often variability in symptoms and impairment across the life span (Evans et al., 2021). It is noteworthy that there are specific features of the disorder among adults that are often identified by practitioners and even noted by the adult patients themselves but are not necessarily delineated in the nosology as outlined in the *DSM-5*. Such symptoms that are core to the presenting symptoms of ADHD may include among others procrastination, a "demoralization syndrome" that includes a persistent sense of failure, poor time management, and, finally, a pervasive tendency to take on more tasks that may be completed on a reasonable basis (Barkley et al., 2008).

### 1.5.1 Disruptive, Impulse-Control, and Conduct Disorders

Oppositional defiant disorder (ODD), conduct disorder (CD), or intermittent explosive disorder are comorbid disorders of ADHD that are most frequently identified among children and adolescents (Evans et al., 2021).

Diagnostic criteria identified in the *DSM-5* (APA, 2013) do indicate that these specific disorders may be employed for adults if criteria are not met for antisocial personality disorder. Because ADHD is frequently a comorbid disorder of antisocial personality disorder, the relevance of these comorbid conditions in adults is fairly apparent. After controlling for chronological age, gender, race, and socioeconomic status (SES), children with ADHD were 12 times more likely to have CD than their typically developing peers. More importantly, for the adult population, the comorbidity of CD is associated with a more severe presentation of ADHD, delinquency, and aggression (The MTA Cooperative Group, 1999). Similar trends have been found for children with ODD, albeit with a less severe presentation of ADHD (Connor & Doerfler, 2008).

Because ODD and CD are frequently comorbid conditions associated with ADHD when diagnosed in childhood and that antisocial personality disorder is frequently a disorder in adulthood following the diagnosis of CD in childhood, the astute clinician should assess for ADHD, particularly when a young adult is suspected of harboring symptoms of ODD or CD. Similarly, the comorbidity of ODD, aggression, and CD in the presence of symptoms associated with ADHD should be carefully assessed as these comorbidities may signal greater severity of ADHD and a more guarded long-term prognosis of the disorder (Connor & Doerfler, 2008).

### 1.5.2  Depressive Disorders

It is noteworthy that individuals with ADHD are three to eight times more likely to experience symptoms of depression than those without the disorder (Larson et al., 2011). When considering some of the symptoms associated with ADHD including a reduced ability to sustain attention, failure to complete tasks, and forgetting to complete daily activities, it also is important to note that such symptoms frequently overlap with mood disorders including major depressive disorder or dysthymic disorder (APA, 2013). In addition, problems with ADHD also frequently include low self-esteem, sleep disturbances, and feelings of restlessness that are also symptomatic among individuals with depressive disorders. Thus, differential diagnosis becomes a formidable task for even the most experienced practitioner. While it is our experience that while many cases of ADHD remain untreated or incorrectly identified, others may believe that they suffer from ADHD when in fact they are experiencing symptoms associated with a mood disorder. For example, during a major depressive episode, many adults may encounter difficulty concentrating at work or being careless at home such as when paying bills. Thus, the wise practitioner must take care to conduct a careful history of the presenting symptoms, particularly for concentration and memory impairments. When related to ADHD, the symptoms are most likely to be chronic from childhood whereas symptoms associated with a mood disorder are apt to become most acute during a major episode and remit between episodes. The differential diagnosis of ADHD and dysthymic disorder is apt to be more complex as symptoms for both disorders are most apt to have persisted over a long period of time.

### 1.5.3 Anxiety Disorders

It has been estimated that approximately 20% of individuals with ADHD also have been diagnosed with a comorbid anxiety disorder and that individuals with ADHD are more likely to experience anxiety than individuals without ADHD (Larson et al., 2011). Symptoms of anxiety include inattention and impaired concentration, which are core symptoms of ADHD. It also is noteworthy that individuals with generalized anxiety disorder may also appear restless, overactive, and fidgety, which are pervasive symptoms among individuals with ADHD. Thus, in attempting to clinically distinguish between the two disorders, the astute practitioner must evaluate whether such symptoms and behaviors are associated with persistent worries and fears that would be consistent with the core symptoms of an anxiety disorder. Identifying the causality and directionality of these symptoms is paramount in differentiating between ADHD and anxiety disorders. For example, among individuals with ADHD, challenges associated with inattention and completing work are likely to result in anxiety and stress. However, among individuals with anxiety disorders, stress and worry may result in an inability to concentrate and thus result in the inability to complete tasks.

### 1.5.4 Trauma- and Stress-Related Disorders

There is some evidence in the extant literature that children with ADHD are at greater risk for sexual abuse (for a review, see Wolfe & Kelly, 2021) and many adults seeking evaluation for ADHD may have experienced traumatic events during childhood thereby making it a challenge to distinguish symptoms due to ADHD from PTSD. Irritability, difficulty concentrating, and sleep disturbances, which are core characteristics of PTSD, also are experienced by many adults with ADHD. Given the remarkable symptom overlap between the two disorders, practitioners would be wise to be cognizant of the symptom presentation for both disorders and to ascertain a complete history as to the emergence of ADHD symptoms and traumatic events. The history is important since ADHD is a disorder with a prolonged course with symptoms that are present from childhood while PTSD typically has a more sudden onset and is typically associated with a specific event (for a review, see Wolfe & Kelly, 2021).

### 1.5.5 Bipolar and Related Disorders

Core symptoms of bipolar disorder may include a high level of energy, restless behavior, impatience, impulsive speech, trouble focusing, and a reduced need for sleep (APA, 2013). These symptoms also mirror those of ADHD and for this reason the differential diagnosis between ADHD and bipolar disorder may be challenging. Of course, full-blown manic episodes that are required for the diagnosis of bipolar I disorder make the identification of bipolar disorder easy to distinguish from ADHD. Specific symptoms that are very specific to bipolar disorder include grandiosity, hypersexuality, decreased need for sleep, and the pervasiveness of mood symptoms (APA, 2013). When clients display a combination of mood instability, impulsivity, irritability, and restlessness, the differential diagnosis of ADHD and bipolar disorder becomes a more formidable task (Fristad & Roley-Roberts, 2021). One distinguishing feature between ADHD and bipolar disorder is elevation of mood, grandiosity, and mood swings that are episodic and dissipate for several weeks and even months such that they alternate with relatively normal mood levels. In differentiating between the two disorders, it cannot be overemphasized how important it is to obtain a detailed history as to onset of the display of symptoms. When symptoms are generally present early in life, follow a chronic course, and are always present, ADHD is likely to be the diagnosis. Alternatively, bipolar disorder frequently manifests itself in late adolescence or young adulthood and is frequently more variable regarding presentation (Fristad & Roley-Roberts, 2021).

### 1.5.6 Personality Disorders

Core symptom features of personality disorders include problems with interpersonal relationships and maladaptive patterns of behavior in the management of these interpersonal relationships. Because of impulsivity and low frustration tolerance, adults with ADHD also may find managing interpersonal relationships and the maintenance of healthy peer relationships challenging. In distinguishing between the diagnoses of borderline personality disorder and ADHD, the retrospective assessment of childhood symptoms is especially important (Fossati et al., 2002). More importantly, individuals with bipolar disorder are more apt to display more severe symptoms of psychopathology than their ADHD counterparts that include but are not limited to preoccupation with suicide, self-mutilation, and feelings of abandonment (Perepletchikova & Nathanson, 2021). While many individuals with antisocial personality disorder have had a history of ADHD during childhood, there are very negative patterns of behavior observed among individuals with antisocial personality disorder that include ongoing rule-violating behaviors and more serious infractions of the law (e.g., theft, ongoing violations of societal laws), as compared to the traditional behaviors observed among individuals with ADHD.

### 1.5.7 Substance-Related and Addictive Disorders

Frequently, impaired concentration that is associated with the sequelae of alcohol and other psychoactive substances (e.g., marijuana, cocaine, stimulants, opiates, nicotine) may mimic or even mask those symptoms associated with ADHD. The literature is clear that individuals with ADHD may abuse substances including tobacco to better manage symptoms associated with ADHD (for a review, see Chung & Bachrach, 2021). Regular use of marijuana may result in problems with motivation, sustaining attention and effort, and problems with cognitive impairment and executive dysfunction that are symptoms most frequently associated with ADHD. In addition, adults who regularly abuse alcohol may display problems associated with attention and concentration, short-term memory, and may make careless errors at home and at work. Thus, a major task for the practitioner is to distinguish between such symptoms that are associated with ADHD or may be the result of substance and alcohol abuse. Frequently, symptoms for both disorders co-occur and it is important to distinguish the symptoms of the two disorders by means of a careful history of the symptoms associated with ADHD. Initially, those symptoms associated with substance abuse should be a priority in clinical practice and subsequently the management of ADHD. Care must be taken when managing ADHD individuals with pharmacotherapy, particularly the stimulants as such agents have potential for abuse and individuals at risk for abuse of other substances are of course at heightened risk for abuse of the stimulants (Subcommittee on Attention-Deficit/Hyperactivity Disorder et al., 2011).

## 1.5.8 Neurodevelopmental, Physical, and Medical Conditions

There are numerous neurodevelopmental disorders whose symptoms mirror those of ADHD and may be frequently comorbid with ADHD. These include specific learning disabilities, language or communication disorders, autism spectrum disorders, seizure disorders, and motor coordination disorders (e.g., stereotypic movement disorder) (for a review, see Evans et al., 2021). Symptoms of ADHD that may overlap with these neurodevelopmental disorders include inattention, disorganization, executive dysfunction, behavioral challenges, and difficulties establishing and maintaining peer relationships (Evans et al., 2021).

Neurodevelopmental disorders are typically identified during childhood when children and adolescents are encountering difficulties in the academic setting or possibly among late adolescents in college. If such disorders are identified during college or in adulthood, differential diagnosis of ADHD from neurodevelopmental disorders may require specialized assessment, which would include a thorough history for the emergence of ADHD symptoms, observations of behaviors across settings and situations, and psychometric or neuropsychological testing to identify the learning disability. Autism spectrum disorders may now be diagnosed as comorbid with ADHD (APA, 2013). It is noteworthy that language and communication disorders also are frequently comorbid with ADHD. Additionally, there are a host of physical and medical conditions whose symptom presentations frequently resemble ADHD in adulthood and such disorders include a variety of sleep disorders (e.g., obstructive sleep apnea, restless leg/periodic limb movement disorder, delayed sleep phase syndrome), acquired traumatic brain injury, hypothyroidism or hyperthyroidism, and visual and hearing impairments. Thus, a careful medical evaluation should always be the standard in the diagnosis of ADHD.

Finally, there are a number of chronic illnesses for which various pharmacotherapies are employed, many of which exert cognitive or behavioral toxicities that frequently mirror symptoms of ADHD (for a review, see Brown, 2018). For example, the therapies most commonly employed to treat cancer (i.e., chemotherapy, radiation therapy), may result in either short-term or long-term central nervous system-related toxicities, frequently referred to as neurocognitive late effects. Such effects may mimic ADHD symptoms, including problems with attention and concentration, memory impairments, and processing speed. In fact, there is a corpus of research to suggest the efficacy of standard pharmacotherapies is similar to those in managing ADHD including the use of stimulant medication (Brown, in press). Of further interest is the finding that the structural central nervous system impairments associated with sickle cell disease are similar to those of individuals with ADHD including abnormalities in the regions of the frontal lobe that manifest in attentional impairments similar to individuals with ADHD. Similarly for those individuals with cancer, the stimulants have proven to have some positive impact on memory and inhibitory control in these individuals and that higher doses of the stimulants enhance parent and teacher ratings of attention and concentration. Finally, for those individuals with asthma, some of the inhalants used by these individuals may have a sympathomimetic untoward effect that produces problems with attention and overactivity.

Thus, in evaluating ADHD in adults, care must be taken to examine neurodevelopmental disorders and physical anomalies including pharmacotherapies employed to treat these anomalies that may mirror symptoms associated with ADHD. In such cases, the clinician must be vigilant in collaborating with primary care colleagues and other medical specialties to rule out for physical disorders or untoward adverse effects associated with their treatment that may be mirroring symptoms associated with ADHD.

## 1.5.9   Environmental and Psychosocial Factors

It is well recognized that ADHD is a constitutional disorder and there is even compelling evidence of a genetic predisposition toward the disorder (Evans et al., 2021). While there is little evidence that environmental factors are etiologic in the disorder, there is no doubt that environmental and psychosocial factors contribute significantly to the expression and exacerbation of behaviors and symptoms associated with inattention, overactivity, and impulsivity. Psychosocial factors may further complicate a diagnosis of ADHD in adulthood that includes past or recent trauma (e.g., neglect, physical or sexual abuse) (Wolfe & Kelly, 2021). It should be noted that recent stressors, including the death of a loved one, loss of a pet, or separation from a significant other may exacerbate symptoms associated with the disorder (Kaplow et al., 2021). This information is important for the clinician as changes or alterations in the environment may likely influence symptom management of the ADHD disorder. While prevalence rates of ADHD among racial-ethnic nonminority and racial-ethnic minority status youth are believed to be generally similar, there is some evidence that Black and Hispanic children are diagnosed at lower rates and, more concerning, are less likely to receive treatment services than their White counterparts (Bussing et al., 2003). However, recent data suggest that although the gap in receiving diagnosis and treatment between Black and White children was lessening, the prevalence rate of diagnosis for Hispanic children is still lower as compared to White children (Bax et al., 2019). Much of this may be attributable to access to mental health care, although knowledge about ADHD and perceptions of ADHD behavior likely impact these data. Differential knowledge may exist about ADHD among individuals of different races and socioeconomic backgrounds (Bax et al., 2019). Thus, when working with culturally diverse populations, clinicians must be aware of these issues and provide appropriate psychoeducation about the disorder.

## 1.6 Comorbidity

ADHD is a pervasive disorder in adult psychiatric outpatient clinics and counseling settings. Comorbid psychiatric disorders are frequently prevalent in a high proportion of adults with ADHD (for a review, see Evans et al., 2021). It has been suggested that nearly 80% of adults with ADHD will present with at least one psychiatric comorbidity (Fischer et al., 2007). It should be noted that the prevalence of comorbidities with ADHD differs significantly between children and adults. In support of this notion, the externalizing behavior problems most frequently co-occur with ADHD in children, while anxiety and mood disorders are the most commonly occurring psychiatric disorders in adults with prevalence rates ranging from 24% to 38% (Larson et al., 2011). Impulse control disorders and substance use disorders also are frequently comorbid with ADHD in adults (Kessler et al., 2006). While the developmental disorders including learning disabilities and the autism spectrum disorders are frequently comorbid with ADHD, there are notable differences in incidence of these disorders between children and adults simply because these disorders are most frequently diagnosed in young children. Alternatively, personality disorders and substance abuse typically emerge in late adolescence or early adulthood. It should be noted that a determination of the true differences in the prevalence of comorbidities is made difficult by specific measurement challenges and variability regarding age of onset of specific conditions. It should be recognized that there are no biomarkers of ADHD available to the practitioner and thus the practitioner is limited to observation, interview, psychiatric history, and rating scales with the latter being limited to specific age ranges such as childhood or adulthood and do not actually assess specific symptoms across the life span.

Different subtypes or presentations of ADHD may confer additional risks for specific comorbidities. For example, findings from an investigation that employed criteria for the *DSM-IV* for ADHD revealed that combined-type ADHD was associated with significantly more lifetime CD, bipolar disorder, and psychosis than the inattentive presentation (Wilens et al., 2009). However, one large-scale investigation of patients at a tertiary referral center revealed few differences in comorbidities between subtypes (Groß-Lesch et al., 2016). It also must be noted that there are significant gender differences in comorbidities in adults with ADHD. Specifically, women with ADHD have been found to have higher rates of mood, anxiety, and eating disorders relative to their male counterparts. Alternatively, substance abuse disorders have been found to be more frequent among males relative to females (45% versus 29%).

## 1.6.1 Oppositional Defiant and Conduct Disorders

The extant literature has long indicated that most children with ADHD from community samples have comorbid ODD or CD and that these comorbidities are more common among males than females (Jensen et al., 2001) with prevalence rates ranging from 42% to 93%. Similarly, the Multimodal Treatment of ADHD (MTA) study found that 39.9% of the sample had comorbid ODD (The MTA Cooperative Group, 1999). Even after controlling for gender, age, race, and SES, children with ADHD were 12 times more likely to have CD than their typically developing peers (Connor & Doerfler, 2008). Given that treatment is similar across each of the three disorders, these comorbidities do not impact treatment planning (Evans et al., 2018), although those with these comorbidities are likely to need additional therapies including anger management, family-based approaches to therapy, as well as strong contingency management approaches across various domains of the individual's life including home, school, and community activities.

Adults with ADHD and a comorbid disruptive or externalizing behavior disorder such as ODD or CD are frequently described as being prone to externalizing blame, frequently arguing, failing to take responsibility for actions, and attempting to control others. Their reactions may include yelling, refusing to adhere to rules, or in more extreme cases escalating to physical aggression or violent behavior. Relative to the precipitant that escalated the conflict, these behaviors are generally characterized as extreme. Adults with ADHD and a comorbid disruptive behavior disorder consistently struggle with self-regulation and have consistently demonstrated this type of reactive behavior over a prolonged period. Adults with ADHD and comorbid conduct disorder are at risk of being involved with the courts and the penal system relative to those individuals with ADHD alone.

## 1.6.2 Depressive Disorders

Various mood disorders such as major depressive disorder and dysthymic disorder can also occur with ADHD. A review of the extant literature reveals that those with ADHD are three to eight times more likely to have symptoms of depression relative to their peers without the disorder (Larson et al., 2011). Findings from national and international surveys of community samples of adults with ADHD reveal a prevalence rate of 38.3% for a co-occurring mood disorder, 18.6% for major depressive disorder, and 12.8% for dysthymia (Fayyad et al., 2017). Moreover, females with ADHD are at greater risk for suicidal ideation and behaviors than those without the disorder (Chronis-Tuscano et al., 2010). It is noteworthy that among youth with ADHD, the onset of depressive symptoms is frequently during young adulthood (Yoshimasu et al., 2016) and is posited to occur due to the cumulative risk associated with ADHD-related impairment coupled with stressful events that interact with genetic risks over the course of time (Blackman et al., 2005). Moreover, those with depression and ADHD frequently experience a more severe and negative course of depression, a greater likelihood of the reoccurrence of depressive episodes, and greater functional impairments than those individuals with depression and without comorbidity of ADHD (for a review, see Evans et al., 2021). Thus, given the severity of the comorbidity of ADHD and depression, it is important that the astute diagnostician assesses for both comorbid conditions when evaluating for ADHD. It also should be noted that there are overlapping symptoms of both disorders and measures to assess depression among comorbid groups are less useful in the identification of depression among those with ADHD than those without the comorbid condition. However, there is available evidence that symptoms of social withdrawal, anhedonia, depressive cognitions, suicidal thoughts, and psychomotor retardation differentiate those with and without comorbid depressive disorders than irritability and concentration problems, which more frequently are associated with symptoms of ADHD (for a review, see Evans et al., 2021).

A common symptom among adults with ADHD where there is significant comorbidity of depressive symptoms is a tendency to inflate the importance of difficult events and to have a dearth of coping resources in response to stress (Evans et al., 2021). These individuals also may exhibit irritability, anger, and social dysfunction relative to their counterparts with ADHD alone. Some individuals with comorbid ADHD and dysthymia have struggled with a chronic low mood and, therefore, may present with low self-esteem and feelings of hopelessness and helplessness thereby being at greater risk for accidents and suicidal behavior than individuals with only one of the disorders. Given the associated characteristics of ADHD and impulsivity, it stands to reason that individuals with comorbid ADHD and depression would be at greater risk for suicidal behavior. Thus, the astute practitioner should always be vigilant for the presence of suicidal ideation, gestures, or behaviors among individuals with comorbid ADHD and depression.

## 1.6.3 Anxiety Disorders

It has been estimated that approximately 17% of those with ADHD have been diagnosed with a comorbid anxiety disorder and that individuals with ADHD are seven times more likely to experience symptoms of anxiety than those without ADHD (Larson et al., 2011). There is clearly an overrepresentation of anxiety disorders among adults with ADHD. In general, studies indicate prevalence rates of 24–43% for generalized anxiety disorder and 52% for a history of overanxious disorder among adults with ADHD (for a review, see Barkley et al., 2008). For example, in the MTA sample, 38% met diagnostic criteria for anxiety disorder. It is particularly noteworthy that those youth with comorbid anxiety disorders were more responsive to behavioral interventions only than were youth with comorbid anxiety disorders and ODD and/or CD thereby suggesting that ADHD youth with comorbid anxiety disorders may benefit in response to a cognitive-behavioral approach (León-Barriera et al., 2022). Thus, the assessment of comorbid anxiety disorders with ADHD is important, as cognitive behavioral therapy (CBT) alone may be sufficient in the management of these individuals. It also is important to note that those with comorbidity of anxiety disorders and externalizing behavioral problems (CD, ODD) benefit from the combination of stimulant medication and behavior management.

Adults with co-occurring anxiety disorders and ADHD are frequently described as "worriers." Unlike adults who have ADHD alone, adults who have both anxiety disorder and ADHD demonstrate explicit symptoms of anxiety, and they evidence undue concerns about their skills and performance in social situations as well as in work settings. These individuals may also display high levels of worrying regarding what people think about what they say or do, and their behavior in activities or at events.

## 1.6.4 Learning Disabilities

Although learning disabilities are primarily identified among children with ADHD, because of their pervasiveness a brief discussion of these comorbidities is warranted here in the discussion of ADHD in adults. It has been estimated that the median prevalence rates of the comorbidity of ADHD and learning disabilities is 47% (DuPaul et al., 2013) with significant variability across studies. The variability has been attributed to the various definitions of learning disabilities (for a review, see Evans et al., 2021). For those in late adolescence or young adulthood, this has implications for performance in college where goals of performance at times exceed the capability of the learner. For example, if a particular subject area requires proficiency in an area of a specific learning disability such as mathematics, a student may need to take advantage of specific accommodations or skills such as tutoring, special study groups, or specialized testing accommodations free from a distracting environment that may be essential to perform in this subject area. Unfortunately, few investigations have examined the efficacy of various approaches amenable to those with comorbid ADHD and learning disabilities. A recent randomized clinical trial examining specific interventions for ADHD and reading disorders found that children benefited from a treatment targeting each specific disorder, although crossover effects were generally not useful for the two comorbidities (Tamm et al., 2017). In addition, a recent investigation by Tannock et al. (2018) obtained similar findings for youth with ADHD and reading disabilities. Unfortunately, no studies could be found that have examined specific treatments for adults with comorbidity of learning disabilities and ADHD. The extant child literature would suggest that for adults with comorbidity of ADHD and learning disabilities, the application of interventions specific to the symptoms of each of the disorders including ADHD (remaining on task, attending to details, completing work without errors) and the specific learning disability are necessary in the management of each condition.

### 1.6.5 Bipolar and Related Disorders

A large systematic evaluation of the association between adult ADHD and bipolar disorder conducted by the National Institute of Mental Health's Systemic Treatment Enhancement Program for Bipolar Disorder has revealed an overall lifetime prevalence rate of 9.5% (14.7% for men; 5.8% for women) (Nierenberg et al., 2005). In addition, findings from a study of lifetime ADHD among individuals with a mood disorder revealed a prevalence rate of 17.6% (McIntyre et al., 2010). It has been noted that ADHD is the second highest comorbid disorder among individuals with bipolar disorders, with those with childhood-onset bipolar disorder being 2.8 times more likely to have comorbid ADHD than those with adolescent onset bipolar disorder (Fristad & Roley-Roberts, 2021). It is important to note that those with comorbidity of ADHD and bipolar disorder tend to exacerbate functioning impairments thereby resulting in increased inpatient hospitalizations (for a review, see Fristad & Roley-Roberts, 2021).

Regarding the management of the comorbid conditions of ADHD and bipolar disorder, there is evidence that the stimulants including methylphenidate and amphetamine salts are efficacious in mitigating symptoms of ADHD without exacerbating mood (Scheffer et al., 2005). Of interest is the finding that the second-generation antipsychotics including both paliperidone and risperidone result in ADHD symptom improvement as well as improvement in manic symptomatology (Joshi et al., 2013). Executive functioning also has been found to improve for those with comorbidity of mood disorders and ADHD following a 3-month trial with omega-3 fatty acids (Vesco et al., 2015). Regarding psychotherapy, group therapy for those with comorbidity of ADHD and bipolar disorder employing a multifamily psycho-educational approach was found to reduce symptoms of ADHD compared to a control group (Fristad et al., 2018). Finally, cognitive remediation has been demonstrated in an open clinical trial of youth with comorbidity of ADHD and bipolar disorder to enhance response inhibition, cognitive flexibility and reduce frustration tolerance. While controlled clinical trials must be conducted to support the veracity of such preliminary findings, the data are promising in the successful management of the comorbidity of ADHD and bipolar disorder.

## 1.6.6 Substance-Related and Addictive Disorders

Substance abuse disorders is one of the most frequent comorbidities found among those with ADHD (Chan et al., 2008). For females with substance use disorders, major depression and trauma syndromes are common (Lotzin et al., 2019), while for males externalizing or disruptive behavior disorders are primarily comorbid with ADHD (Roberts et al., 2007). It is noteworthy that ADHD poses an especially salient risk factor for the development of substance use disorders and may also impact recovery from prolonged drug and alcohol abuse. The prevalence of comorbid substance abuse disorder among adults with persistent ADHD has been estimated at 47% or higher (Bukstein, 2012). Adults with ADHD are at greatest risk for abusing drugs and alcohol, using substances at earlier ages, and developing one or more substance use disorders than their same gender peers without ADHD (Chung & Bachrach, 2021). In fact, the presence of ADHD poses a twofold increase in the propensity to develop substance abuse disorders across the life span (for a review, see Chung & Bachrach, 2021). Some individuals with ADHD may use substances as a means of medicating their ADHD symptoms. Research has identified several variables that account for increased risk of substance abuse disorders in adults with ADHD, which include severity of the ADHD symptoms, comorbidities of ODD and conduct disorder, temperament characteristics, family history of comorbid substance abuse and ADHD, and finally male gender (Chung & Bachrach, 2021).

Cigarette smoking and nicotine dependence have been demonstrated to be highly prevalent among adults with ADHD. Interestingly, it is noteworthy that those individuals with ADHD are more likely to become regular smokers, begin smoking at an earlier age, to smoke more heavily, and have more difficulty in quitting smoking (for a review, see Chung & Bachrach, 2021). In addition, Biederman and associates (2012) found that over one fourth of adults with ADHD were nicotine dependent relative to 11% of controls. Of interest also is the finding that individuals with ADHD may also consume caffeine in greater quantities than those individuals who do not have symptoms associated with ADHD (for a review, see Evans et al., 2021).

## 1.6.7 Personality Disorders

Personality disorders frequently co-occur among adults with ADHD (for a review, see Perepletchikova & Nathanson, 2021). Results from the National Epidemiologic Survey on Alcohol and Related Conditions reported comorbid personality disorders in 62.8% of adults with ADHD relative to 20.5%

in the general population (Bernardi et al., 2012). It is noteworthy that those with reactive temperament, characterized by being emotionally frustrated in response to stress, symptoms associated with ADHD, may be at higher risk for developing borderline personality disorder, particularly if they experience peer victimization (Haltigan & Vaillancourt, 2016). In a large longitudinal investigation of 2,450 girls, findings indicated that elevated levels of emotionality and low levels of sociability predicted greater risk in the development of borderline personality symptoms in later adolescence and early adulthood (Stepp et al., 2014). Borderline personality disorder is a frequent comorbid disorder among adults with ADHD (Weiner et al., 2019). Finally, the reported rates of comorbidity for antisocial personality disorder and ADHD ranges from 13% to 44% (Torgersen et al., 2006).

### 1.6.8 Sleep–Wake Disorders

It has been estimated that between 25% and 50% of caregivers of children with ADHD have noted the presence of sleep problems in their children, which include difficulties initiating and maintaining sleep (for a review, see Graef & Byars, 2021). Similarly, sleep problems are a pervasive comorbid condition among adults with ADHD. Other problems associated with comorbid ADHD and sleep–wake disorders include sleep-disordered breathing, poor sleep efficiency, increased sleep latency, and decreased total sleep time relative to healthy comparison controls (for a review, see Graef & Byars, 2021). Symptoms associated with sleep disorders in adults include difficulty falling and remaining asleep, shorter sleep duration, and difficulties remaining alert throughout the day. Even when they obtain an acceptable amount of sleep during the previous night, adults with ADHD also may exhibit difficulties with awakening. The difficulties may have ramifications for functional capacity throughout the day as these individuals are frequently late for work and have difficulties remaining alert throughout the day, particularly when they must sit for long periods of time or perform rote or routine tasks. Due to the variability of objectively measuring sleep–wake patterns among those with ADHD, there have been conflicting findings in this literature. Practitioners also may misdiagnose a sleep disorder as ADHD or even miss sleep disorders among individuals diagnosed with ADHD. Findings from an investigation that compared adults with narcolepsy, idiopathic hypersomnia, and ADHD found a high percentage of symptom overlap, which the investigators of the study attributed to potential misdiagnosis of ADHD among adults (Oosterloo et al., 2006).

It also should be noted that those with ADHD are more apt to exhibit inadequate sleep hygiene due to difficulties in settling into a routine bedtime and resisting bedtime routines and stalling when it comes to sleep routines. In addition, those with fragmented or inadequate sleep are more likely to exhibit daytime behaviors that resemble ADHD including hyperactivity, impulsivity, inattention, and disruptive behavior. Because sleep deprivation or disturbances may give rise to or exacerbate ADHD symptoms, proper evaluation of sleep deprivation or disturbances in adults with ADHD is warranted. Finally, all ADHD assessments should include questions regarding sleep routines, daytime sleepiness, patterns and persistence of sleep difficulties, and education regarding sleep hygiene.

It is believed that the interaction between sleep-wake disorders and ADHD is a reflection of shared neurobiological pathways (Owens, 2008). In considering these issues, Graef and Byars (2021) advise that the astute practitioner consider how arousal and sleep regulation may interact with environmental and physiological influences including stimulant medication in the delay of sleep onset (for a review, see Graef & Byars, 2021). Clearly the association between sleep disorders and ADHD requires ongoing assessment and specific intervention within a neurobiological and environmental framework (for a review, see Graef & Byars, 2021). For this reason, the management of individuals with ADHD and sleep disturbances should include a combination of psychoeducation regarding sleep hygiene in combination with sleep schedules.

## 1.7 Diagnostic Procedures and Documentation

The diagnosis of ADHD in adults can be particularly challenging and therefore a trained professional with specific training in ADHD as well as the identification of other psychiatric disorders should make the diagnosis. This might include clinical psychologists, adult psychiatrists, clinical social workers, primary care providers, or neurologists. The use of a systematic approach in gathering data across all sources and settings from multiple informants is imperative in accurately diagnosing ADHD. The diagnosis of adult ADHD is often made based on history of childhood symptoms as well as current behavior and level of global functioning (e.g., work, social relationships, marriage) in the past 6 months. Therefore, the first step for practitioners in the diagnostic process is to conduct a comprehensive clinical interview with the individual and, if possible, other relevant informants, to obtain information about primary presenting symptoms and problems. This evaluation should include a personal and family history obtained through interviews and a review of medical records, and psychological test results if these are in fact available. Because adults may be unable to accurately recall early symptoms, obtaining collateral information from a parent, sibling, or other family member is helpful in establishing a childhood history of ADHD. The review of medical records is important as there may be indications of hearing, vision, or medical problems (e.g., hyperthyroidism). The professional should evaluate whether the adult meets symptomatic criteria for ADHD according to *DSM-5-TR* or *ICD-10* criteria. This is best accomplished by asking specific questions about ADHD symptoms while also focusing on gathering information about the onset, frequency, and severity of such symptoms. This process also may include the use of rating forms across settings and situations.

> **Practitioners should gather data across sources from multiple informants when diagnosing ADHD**

> **No single attentional, educational, medical, or neurological test can reliably identify ADHD**

During the initial comprehensive interview, the clinician also should accumulate information that will rule out other possible causes of ADHD symptoms that might include symptoms of anxiety or depression, a situational stressor such as a divorce or the death of a loved one, and medical disorders that may affect central nervous system dysfunction such as temporal lobe seizures or hypo- or hyperthyroidism. The clinician also should seek to determine whether the home or work environments are stressful, chaotic, or lack structure and, if possible, the adult should be observed in these various settings. Such information may provide data about possible stressors that may be causing or exacerbating symptoms and may have important treatment implications.

Another important step in the assessment process is to determine whether other comorbid conditions or disorders (see Section 1.6) may coexist with ADHD. In the case of coexisting conditions, the clinician should determine which disorder is primary or secondary to better inform treatment decisions. In addition, the clinician should generate alternative hypotheses for the differential diagnostic process. Further, it is important that the clinician determine individual and family strengths and assets that may be especially relevant when developing the treatment plan to best provide support for the affected individual. As is true with the diagnosis of any mental health disorder, clinicians should also consider how cultural factors influence symptom presentation.

> Practitioners should gather data from a variety of measures, sources, and across several settings

One of the most important aspects of the diagnostic process for ADHD is that practitioners obtain information from a variety of measures and instruments (e.g., structured interviews, clinician-rated and self-report rating scales, objective testing), from a variety of sources (e.g., family members or mental health clinicians that work with the adult), and across several settings (e.g., at home, work). Different strategies for gathering this important information from the adult and other relevant informants are described in greater detail in Sections 1.7.1–1.7.5. It is worth mentioning again that most of the diagnostic instruments and rating scales in this section were developed based on *DSM-IV-TR* criteria for the diagnosis of ADHD and, given some of the more recent changes in diagnostic nomenclature, the practitioner may encounter some ambiguities in the diagnostic process.

## 1.7.1 Diagnostic Interviews

> Structured and semistructured instruments help define normal and abnormal behavior

Structured and semistructured interviews conducted with the adult and other informants (e.g., family members) represent a top-down approach to assessment and are most consistent with the criteria listed in the *DSM*. The purpose of using these structured and semistructured instruments in the assessment process is to establish limits between typically occurring and atypical behavior. This approach is frequently referred to as a categorical approach because it results in a yes/no decision for diagnosis. Although these interviews are considered the gold standard by psychologists and psychiatrists for assessing psychopathology (Nordgaard et al., 2012), ADHD is not included in some of the commonly used structured psychiatric interviews for adults. In addition, the use of these structured interviews requires significant training, and is time intensive and costly, making them difficult to implement in busy clinical settings. The Kiddie Schedule for Affective Disorders and Schizophrenia for School-Age Children (Ambrosini, 2000) is a semistructured psychiatric interview that was designed for use with children but has been used with some success for adults (Biederman et al., 2006). The Diagnostic Interview for ADHD in Adults is a semistructured interview for ADHD in adults (Kooij & Francken, 2010). The Mini-International Neuropsychiatric Interview (MINI) – Plus contains a module for ADHD that has questions related to child and adult behavior (Lecrubier et al., 1997) and covers the current core ADHD symptoms. The MINI-Plus also allows for the assessment of a broad range of psychopathology, which is important when considering differential diagnosis. The Conners' Adult ADHD Diagnostic Interview for DSM-IV (Epstein et al., 2001) also has proven useful for clinicians seeking to affirm a diagnosis of ADHD in adults.

### 1.7.2 Rating Scales

The use of standardized symptom or behavioral rating scales from the clinician (clinician rated), adult (self-rating), and family members (spouse, partner, parent, sibling), close friends, or coworkers is recommended in the ADHD assessment process (for examples, see Table 1). These rating scales represent an empirically based bottom-up approach to assessing symptoms and are referred to as a dimensional approach to the assessment of ADHD because the scores do not represent a clear delineation of the presence or absence of the disorder. Unlike structured psychiatric interviews, behaviors or symptoms are assessed along a continuum from normal to atypical in which the goal is to assess how the adult compares to peers in a similar age range. When evaluating to affirm the diagnosis of ADHD in an adult, there are several clinician-rated scales that demonstrate strong psychometric properties. These scales include the Adult ADHD Clinical Diagnostic Scale v.1.2 (Kessler et al., 2007), Brown Executive Function/Attention Scales (Brown, 2018), and the Conners' Adult ADHD Rating Scale (CAARS; La Malfa et al., 2008). The use of self-report behavior rating scales also are important in the diagnostic process. These include the Barkley Adult ADHD Rating Scale-IV (BAARS-IV; Barkley, 2011), the Brown Adult ADHD Scale (Brown & Gammon, 1991), the Conners' Adult ADHD Rating Scales: Self-Report (Conners et al., 1999), the Adult ADHD Self-Report Scale (ASRS; Kessler et al., 2005), and the Wender Utah Rating Scale (McCann et al., 2000). In addition, the BAARS-IV offers an "other-report" form that can be completed by a spouse, parent, or sibling. It should be noted, however, that there has been a large body of research that has cast doubt on the use of self-report ratings for children with ADHD. Whether the use of self-report data for the identification of ADHD among adults yields strong reliability with adults relative to pediatric populations remains to be addressed.

*Standardized rating scales are very important in the ADHD assessment process*

### Table 1
### Adult ADHD Rating Scales

| Rating scale | Description |
| --- | --- |
| **Clinician-rated scale** | |
| Adult ADHD Clinical Diagnostic Scale (ACDS) | Semistructured interview to evaluate current adult symptoms of ADHD. |
| Brown Attention-Deficit Disorder Scale (BADDS) | Four-point symptom frequency rating scale. Focuses mostly on symptoms of inattention. |
| Conners' Adult ADHD Diagnostic Interview (CAA-DID) | Eighteen-item scale that contains separate queries for childhood (retrospective) and adult ADHD symptoms. |
| **Self-report behavior rating scale** | |
| Barkley Adult ADHD Rating Scale-IV | Assesses age of onset of symptoms and associated impairment across settings. |
| Brown Adult ADHD Rating Scale | Four-point frequency rating scale that assesses cognitive symptoms associated with difficulty initiating and maintaining optimal concentration and arousal. |
| Copeland Symptom Checklist for Adult ADHD | Sixty-three questions that measure a broad range of cognitive, emotional, and social symptoms on a three-point severity scale. |
| Adult ADHD Self-Report Scale (ASRS) | Frequency-based scale that matches the 18 items in the *DSM-IV*. Includes situational "context" for describing symptoms. |
| Wender Utah Rating Scale | Retrospective five-point severity scale of childhood ADHD symptoms. |
| **Informant symptom inventories** | |
| Barkley Adult ADHD Rating Scale-IV | Assesses age of onset of symptoms and associated impairment across settings. |

> It is important that practitioners evaluate for symptoms and their level of impairment

It is recommended that clinicians not simply assess for symptoms, but also evaluate the level of functional impairment related to such symptoms. Important domains of impairment that should be assessed include family interactions, peer relationships, and vocational performance. One way to evaluate these domains is through direct observation or functional behavioral assessments. However, these observations or assessments are typically more difficult to complete with adult patients. Therefore, rating scales such as the BAARS-IV: Other-Report can be used to assess the degree of ADHD impairment across different settings such as home and work. Again, it must be underscored that to qualify for a diagnosis of ADHD, the adult must evidence some degree of functional impairment in at least one setting as well as a sufficient number of symptoms for the disorder.

## 1.7.3 Psychoeducational Testing

Psychoeducational testing may be considered for young adults struggling with academic performance at college or for adults with a suspected learning disability not yet diagnosed that is impacting work performance. In general, the goal of this type of assessment is to identify the factors contributing to these problems and subsequently recommend appropriate strategies and accommodations that will assist the adult in compensating for these challenges. These tests often assess cognitive strengths and weaknesses, academic skills, information processing, attention or memory challenges, psychological problems such as anxiety or depression, or some other source or combination of factors. Tests of intelligence and achievement should be administered where there is indication that a learning disability may be involved. It is important to underscore that psychoeducational tests are not sufficiently sensitive or specific in identifying ADHD: Rather they are useful in the identification of other comorbidities such as developmental deficits including specific learning disabilities or intellectual disability.

*Tests of intelligence and achievement may help identify a comorbid learning disorder*

## 1.7.4 Neuropsychological Testing

No single neuropsychological test can reliably identify ADHD in an adult or predict response to treatment for ADHD such as stimulant medication. However, performance on a combination of neuropsychological tests may yield useful information and therefore comprise an important component of diagnosis of symptoms for ADHD (i.e., the identification of attentional problems) as well as other comorbidities. In many circumstances the test results also may help clinicians identify learning issues that may be relevant for the college setting or the workplace. Cognitive impairments in adults with ADHD that are often assessed by neuropsychological testing include selective attention, memory, reaction time and information processing speed, motor speed and visuomotor ability, and executive functions.

Neuropsychological tests that measure attention include the Tests of Variables of Attention (Greenberg & Waldman, 1993), go/no-go tasks, the rapid visual information processing task, and the Conners' Continuous Performance Test – third edition (CPT-3; Conners & Staff, 2014). Other neuropsychological assessments often include tests of verbal working memory, such as the Digit Span Test (e.g., Wechsler, 2008), the California Verbal Learning Test – third edition (Delis et al., 2017), and the Wechsler Memory Scale – fourth edition (Wechsler, 2009). Important tests that measure mental flexibility, working memory, and/or executive function include the Wisconsin Card Sorting Test (Berg, 1948), the Stroop Color-Word Interference Test (Golden, 1978), the Rey–Osterrieth Complex Figure (Osterrieth, 1944), and the Delis-Kaplin Executive Function System (Delis et al., 2001). Finally, tests that evaluate multiple abilities include the Developmental NEuroPSYchological Assessment – second edition (Korkman et al., 2007) and the Cambridge Neuropsychological Test Automated Battery

*Performance on neuropsychological tests provide useful information in the diagnosis of ADHD*

(Sahakian et al., 1988). Some of these neuropsychological tests are discussed in greater detail in Chapter 3.

It is important to note that some individuals may be motivated to obtain a diagnosis of ADHD to secure external incentives such as access to medication (for personal use or resale) or workplace accommodations. Therefore, tests of malingering, such as the Test of Memory Malingering, may be included as part of the neuropsychological battery to evaluate for the presence of exaggerated performance or an individual seeking to "fake bad."

### 1.7.5 Laboratory Testing

> Laboratory and other testing is not indicated in the context of an unremarkable medical history for ADHD

The diagnosis of ADHD is based on clinical evaluation. Laboratory, physiologic, radiologic, or neurological testing is not indicated in the context of an unremarkable medical history for ADHD. While evoked potentials, genetic testing, and functional brain imaging have been used in research studies of adults with ADHD, no indication exists for the use of these procedures in the clinical setting because these tests still lack well-defined clinical utility. Quantitative electroencephalography measures have demonstrated some validity, but questions remain about their utility and feasibility for diagnostic use for adults with ADHD.

# 2

# Theories and Models of ADHD in Adults

## 2.1 Neurobiological Factors in ADHD

### 2.1.1 Genetic Contributions

ADHD is among the most heritable of psychiatric disorders. Findings from 37 twin studies of ADHD or measures of inattentiveness and hyperactivity revealed a mean heritability of 74% (Faraone & Larsson, 2019). A recent study of monozygotic and dizygotic twins, full siblings, and maternal and paternal half-siblings found a mean heritability estimate of approximately 80% (Chen et al., 2017). Although the extant literature has demonstrated a strong genetic component for susceptibility to ADHD, studies aimed at identifying specific genes that may be associated with the disorder reveal, at the individual level, effects that are very small (Faraone & Larsson, 2019). Genetic studies generally suggest variations in dopamine receptor genes (Kooij et al., 2010). For example, studies among adults with ADHD identified reduced availability of the $D_2/D_3$ dopamine receptor subtypes, which also is associated with symptoms of inattention (Cortese, 2012). In addition, genetic abnormalities in noradrenergic and serotonergic transporters have been identified in several molecular genetic investigations of children and adults with ADHD (Cortese, 2012). However, the many candidate genes identified to date account for only about 30% of the variance in heritability for ADHD in twin studies (Faraone & Larsson, 2019).

Studies have failed to provide a definitive genetic explanation for why some, but not all, individuals diagnosed with ADHD as children continue to meet diagnostic criteria into adulthood. Some evidence regarding the natural history of the disorder points to differences in heritability for ADHD between children and adults. For example, although twin studies in children have identified a 76% heritability index for ADHD, this value drops to 30–40% among adult twins (Franke et al., 2012). However, when multiple sources of information are applied, the heritability of clinically diagnosed adult ADHD and child ADHD is very similar. Some evidence suggests that ADHD that persists into adulthood may represent an especially heritable form of the disorder that involves different alleles and genes. Linkage studies have identified *LPHN3* and *CDH13* as novel genes associated with ADHD across the life span (Franke et al., 2012). Although research into the genetics of ADHD is advancing, it is still difficult to draw definitive conclusions regarding a genetic etiology for adult ADHD. As is true of many complex psychiatric disorders featuring a genetic component, ADHD likely arises from a combination of genes of weak or moderate effect interacting with environmental factors (Faraone & Larsson, 2019).

### 2.1.2 Neurological Factors

Although the specific pathophysiology of ADHD has yet to be established, studies have identified numerous neurological correlates (Cortese, 2012). Key areas of interest in the pathophysiology of ADHD involve fronto-striatal areas, particularly the fronto-dorsal striatal circuit and the fronto-ventral striatal circuit (Shen et al., 2020). Notably, executive functions such as inhibitory control, selective attention, goal-directed behavior, focus, and decision making are heavily dependent on these areas of the brain (Cortese, 2012). Although some controversy surrounds this body of research, numerous well-designed studies have identified ADHD-related brain morphology in very young children that remain stable throughout development and cannot be accounted for by psychopharmacological interventions (Cortese, 2012).

The diagnosis of ADHD in adults is associated with widespread micro- and macrostructural changes (Gehricke et al., 2017). Studies that have examined relationships between ADHD and brain structure in children with ADHD relative to their normally developing peers demonstrate reductions in overall brain volume with localized volumetric decreases in the right frontal cortex, corpus callosum, caudate nucleus, and cerebellar vermis (Cortese, 2012). Neuroimaging studies focused on ADHD among adults are less robust than the child ADHD literature. Of the available studies employing magnetic imaging, findings reveal dysfunction in the superior longitudinal fasciculus and corticolimbic areas in young adults with ADHD (Gehricke et al., 2017).

Functional magnetic resonance imaging (fMRI) techniques also have made important contributions to our current understanding of ADHD. Meta-analyses of fMRI studies of executive functions indicate that ADHD patients have multisystem impairments in several right- and left-hemispheric dorsal, ventral, and medial fronto-cingulo-striato-thalamic and fronto-parieto-cerebellar networks (Rubia, 2018). These impairments impact cognitive control, attention, timing, and working memory. Findings from fMRI research focused on adults diagnosed with ADHD generally are in accordance with results from studies of ADHD among children.

> Evidence implicates abnormalities in dopamine pathways in individuals with ADHD

There is a growing body of research that has examined the neurochemical properties of ADHD including abnormalities in the dopaminergic, adrenergic, serotonergic, and cholinergic pathways (Cortese, 2012). The most compelling evidence implicating abnormalities in dopamine pathways in individuals with ADHD is that stimulant medications used to manage the symptoms of the disorder increase availability of dopamine in the brain. Some evidence exists that stimulants also increase available levels of norepinephrine; however, this research is less developed due in part to a lack of effective norepinephrine tracers (Cortese, 2012). Additional support for hypoactive dopaminergic systems in individuals with ADHD has been demonstrated in studies revealing reduced volume and blood flow in brain regions that are dense in dopamine (e.g., the caudate nucleus, globus pallidus, and striatum).

Several theoretical models have been developed to explain relationships between dopaminergic abnormalities and symptoms of ADHD (Sagvolden et al., 2005; Tripp & Wickens, 2008). The premise of the first model, a dynamic developmental theory, is that dopamine serves a regulatory function in the brain and is crucial to learning processes through its role in the brain's reward system (Sagvolden et al., 2005). Individuals with ADHD experience hypoactive dopamine release during the learning process, thereby resulting in a shorter available time for associating behavior with consequences. In accordance with this theory of ADHD, abnormal learning results in problems with extinguishing negative behaviors, difficulty with delayed rewards, impulsivity, inattention, and disinhibition (Sagvolden et al., 2005). In a slightly different theoretical model developed to explain relationships between dopamine and ADHD, Tripp and Wickens (2008) posit that children with ADHD fail to develop *anticipatory* dopamine release that signals reinforcing events. As such, children with ADHD are not reinforced for participating in on-task behaviors, and hyperactivity and impulsivity result from unusual sensitivity to delayed reinforcement (Tripp & Wickens, 2008). Although both theories suggest that abnormal learning processes are associated with ADHD, the precise role of dopamine in this process has not yet been clearly defined. In addition, some researchers suggest that ADHD among adults represents a distinct population with unique neurobiological features that are not yet clearly understood (Schneider et al., 2006).

**Several theories suggest that impaired learning processes are associated with ADHD**

Another theory of ADHD that encompasses neurobiological findings is the developmental theory provided by Halperin and Schulz (2006). This theory suggests that variability in development of the prefrontal cortex may explain differential diminishment of symptoms with age. Drawing on findings revealing inconsistent executive function deficits and neuroimaging data in adults with ADHD, these experts cast doubt on prefrontal cortical abnormalities and their *causal* role in ADHD. Rather, Halperin and Schwartz theorize that prefrontal cortical development compensates for early abnormalities in other areas of the brain that have resulted in arousal mechanisms that are simply not effective. These experts argue that variations in ADHD "recovery" are essentially variations in the degree to which prefrontal cortical development has corrected early abnormalities in brain structure and connectivity.

Structural, functional, and neurochemical research in ADHD continues to make significant advances but is still considered in the early stages. As a result, many findings have been contradicted or inconsistently replicated (Halperin & Schulz, 2006). This is not surprising since the brain basis for ADHD appears to involve multiple large-scale, highly complex networks and systems that are difficult to investigate simultaneously (Cortese, 2012). Moreover, the heterogeneity of ADHD symptoms and varying developmental presentations complicate efforts to identify a clear neurobiological etiology of the disorder (Drechsler et al., 2020).

### 2.1.3 Cognitive Determinants

Although stable neurocognitive patterns can be identified in individuals with ADHD, it is a disorder in which neuropsychological strengths and deficits may vary widely (Guo et al., 2021). Findings from a recent systematic review suggest that clinicians focus more on measures of reaction time variability, intelligence and achievement, vigilance, working memory, and response inhibition more when conducting evaluations, and direct less attention to measures of reaction time, set shifting, and decision making (Pievsky & McGrath, 2018). However, there is still controversy about the utility of neuropsychological testing in diagnosing adults with ADHD. Marshall and colleagues (2021) argue that there is limited diagnostic utility of both individual tests and batteries of cognitive tests, but also acknowledge this recommendation should be considered in the context of major study design limitations.

> Russell Barkley's model is a useful formulation of ADHD

In response to neurocognitive deficits observed in individuals with ADHD, Barkley (1997) developed the unifying theory to help explain the etiology and course of ADHD. This theory argues that executive dysfunction – and, specifically, poor behavioral inhibition – is the central and core deficit of ADHD. Barkley defines behavioral inhibition as a threefold process of inhibiting initial responses to an event, discontinuing an ongoing response, and interference control. In accordance with this model, fundamental difficulties with impulse control give rise to difficulties with more complex behaviors including self-regulation of affect, motivation, and arousal; motor control; working memory; and self-directed or self-regulatory speech. As such, poor behavioral inhibition results in acting impulsively, perseverating, and lacking self-control among individuals with ADHD. In response to more recent research findings, Barkley and Fischer (2010) later added deficits in self-awareness and self-directed attention as core facets of executive dysfunction that compromise the ability of individuals with ADHD to engage in goal-directed behaviors. Barkley's unifying theory has been highly influential in the field of ADHD research, leading to numerous investigations of executive dysfunctions in this population. However, questions of how and why executive deficits occur in adults with ADHD, and whether prefrontal cortical abnormalities represent the primary source of ADHD symptoms, and whether these symptoms persist throughout the life span, remain a major focus of further investigation.

## 2.2 Environmental Risk Factors

Although the precise etiology of ADHD has yet to be determined, many studies indicate that genetics and neurobiological factors account for the majority of risk in susceptibility to the disorder (Faraone & Larsson, 2019). In addition to inherited factors, research suggests that environmental risk factors likely contribute to the development of ADHD (Silva & Ibilola, 2021). Because ADHD is a childhood-onset disorder, many of the environmental risk factors for ADHD occur prenatally or during early childhood. These factors include pregnancy and delivery complications, maternal smoking during pregnancy, toxins, dietary factors, and psychosocial adversity (Thapar et al., 2013). While these factors are not necessarily causal, they are associated with or may exacerbate a constitutional predisposition to the disorder or its symptoms.

## 2.2.1 Biological Adversity Factors

Teratogens are drugs, substances, or conditions crossing the placenta that negatively impact developing brain tissue and can result in long-lasting behavioral and learning impairments for children exposed while in the womb. Research findings suggest that maternal obesity, overweight, preeclampsia, hypertension, acetaminophen use, and smoking during pregnancy, as well as childhood asthma and eczema were associated with the development of ADHD in their offspring (Kim et al., 2020). However, maternal obesity, overweight, and smoking during pregnancy were not found to be specific risk factors in familial studies, indicating that other factors (e.g., genetics or other environmental factors) may better explain these associations. Some evidence also suggests that maternal psychological stress during pregnancy, particularly during the third trimester, may be associated with increased risk of ADHD in offspring (Manzari et al., 2019). The authors noted several limitations with the current data on maternal stress and ADHD, which prevented them from drawing more definitive conclusions on this relationship.

Substance use also has been implicated in ADHD development. For example, heavy alcohol use and binge drinking during pregnancy have consistently been associated with ADHD symptoms in progeny (Yolton et al., 2014). Although low to moderate prenatal alcohol exposure has not been found to increase risk for ADHD (San Martin Porter et al., 2019), some research indicates that more complex attentional skills (e.g., shifting attention) may be negatively impacted by even low levels of prenatal alcohol exposure (Pyman et al., 2021). Preliminary findings also suggest associations between prenatal cocaine, methamphetamine, and heroin exposure and development of ADHD symptoms (Yolton et al., 2014).

Regarding perinatal factors, research suggests that pregnancy and labor/delivery complications, including premature birth and low birth weight, increase the risk for symptoms of ADHD (Sciberras et al., 2017). This relationship was more robust for very preterm (gestational age of less than 32 weeks) and low birth weight newborns (less than 5 lbs, 8 oz (2.49 kg) at birth; Franz et al., 2018). However, heterogeneity in study design, common for much of the literature on the association between prenatal (e.g., Manzari et al., 2019) and perinatal factors (Franz et al., 2018) and risk for ADHD, prevented the examination of mediators and potential pathways to explain this relationship.

Postnatal factors implicated in the development of ADHD include severe traumatic brain injury (Asarnow et al., 2021) and infections (Pedersen et al., 2020). Some research also suggests that postnatal exposure to secondhand smoke may be a risk factor for ADHD in children (Huang et al., 2021). Notably, findings from these research studies did not identify mechanisms to explain this association.

### 2.2.2 Environmental Toxins

The results from several studies indicated that some toxins and organic pollutants are associated with symptoms of ADHD, including prenatal exposure to polychlorinated biphenyls (i.e., manufactured compounds that are highly resistant to extreme temperature and pressure) and postnatal exposure to organophosphate pesticides and lead (Thapar et al., 2013; Yolton et al., 2014).

### 2.2.3 Food Additives/Dietary Factors

Systematic studies that examined food additives and dietary factors have only found associations, and not causal relationships, with ADHD. Specific nutritional deficiencies (e.g., iron, zinc, iodine, polyunsaturated fatty acids) and additives (e.g., sugar, artificial food colorings) have all been linked to ADHD (Del-Ponte et al., 2019; Thapar et al., 2013). Although some study findings suggest there may be dietary interventions that could reduce ADHD symptoms, research to date has not included randomized control trials to support any specific dietary intervention (Breda et al., 2022).

## 2.3 Psychosocial Adversity Factors

Psychosocial adversity factors have been demonstrated to increase the risk of ADHD or even exacerbate the severity of symptoms of the disorder. In a seminal investigation on this issue, Rutter and colleagues (1975) demonstrated that the aggregate of six risk factors within a family, rather than the presence of any single factor, contributed to psychopathology. Factors included marital discord, low social class, large family size, paternal criminality, maternal mental disorder, and foster care placement. In particular, SES and ethnic minority status have been associated with lower rates of treatment adherence (Fernandez & Eyberg, 2009). Moreover, in the MTA study, a significant association between economic difficulties and barriers to treatment adherence have been clearly demonstrated (Rieppi et al., 2002). Thus, in their work with disadvantaged clients, the practitioner must be acutely aware of the impact of SES on parent engagement with treatment and must take active initiatives to assist families in overcoming such treatment barriers.

Regarding racial and ethnic minority status, while no differences in prevalence rates have been demonstrated, there is some compelling evidence to suggest that African Americans and Latino individuals are identified as ADHD at lower rates and less likely to receive services relative to their majority counterparts (for review see, Evans et al., 2018). In addition, African Americans are less likely than their majority counterparts to be informed about the etiology of the disorder and may be more likely to attribute the ADHD disorder to genetic issues. Thus, the influence of culture on knowledge of the disorder is especially important in working with minority families. It also should be noted that minority families and particularly those who are overrepresented among lower SES groups encounter myriad barriers to accessing and completing treatment.

It also is noteworthy that family-environment variables may serve as salient risk factors for ADHD (Froehlich et al., 2011). For example, Knopik and colleagues (2005) have demonstrated that alcohol abuse increased the likelihood of an ADHD diagnosis. Additional studies have revealed that family adversity, low-income status, and conflict/parent–child hostility are associated with ADHD (for a review, see Thapar et al., 2013). It is important to point out that psychosocial adversity factors are associated with psychopathology in general and are not specific to ADHD.

## 2.4 Interactions Between Neurobiological, Environmental, and Psychosocial Adversity Factors

It should be noted that ADHD is a clinically heterogeneous disorder among children and adults and there are no specific risk factors that provide an explanation to the etiology of the disorder. Barkley (2020) has concluded that biological factors or aberrations in brain development are most likely associated with the etiology of ADHD. Evidence from family, twin, adoption, genome, and candidate gene search studies implicate genetics as the strongest risk factor in the development of ADHD. These genetic factors seem to be a more viable predictor than those of environmental agents or psychosocial factors. Brain studies of individuals with ADHD suggest delayed maturation in brain development, poor connectivity, and less brain activity in the prefrontal regions of the brain. It should be no surprise that these areas of the brain have been demonstrated to be involved in those areas in which individuals with ADHD exhibit their greatest challenges including executive functioning and self-control, resistance to distraction as well as activity level (Barkley, 2020). This altered brain development and functioning may likely be due to different genetic variations in brain development. In support of this notion, Nigg (2000) has suggested that an understanding of the etiology of ADHD will likely be gleaned from an investigation of gene–environment interactions. In this case, the environment includes both biological and psychosocial events that negatively impact the development of the child.

While much of the evidence to date suggests a genetic basis to ADHD, there is some research to suggest that a smaller percentage of individuals with the disorder acquire ADHD due to acquired injuries of the developing brain including toxins consumed prenatally or following birth. While some have offered the explanation that genetics and environment differentially impact neurobiology, which in turn expresses itself as symptoms of ADHD, research over the past decade has clearly underscored biological determinants of the disorder. Of course, stressors associated with low SES and cultural differences that might impact treatment adherence all have been posited. It remains the task of future research methodologies to assist us in fully comprehending the etiology and expression of ADHD including molecular genetics, epigenetics, and neuroimaging.

# 3

# Diagnosis and Treatment Indications

Many adults refer themselves for evaluations after their children receive an ADHD diagnosis, if they recognize similar disturbances that they themselves have endured. Additional referral sources include family members (such as a spouse or caregiver), the adult's primary care physician, or a medical specialist. Adults are referred for an ADHD evaluation for a variety of reasons that may include long-standing challenges with organizing, planning and time management, poor job performance, and impaired social and family relationships. Adults with ADHD change employers more frequently, have less job satisfaction and fewer occupational achievements, encounter more difficulty completing assignments, have more difficulty working independently, and experience more unstable long-term relationships (Barkley & Benton, 2021).

Accurately diagnosing ADHD among adults can be especially challenging because symptoms commonly associated with ADHD can also be related to a variety of other mental health conditions (e.g., depression, anxiety, bipolar disorder). Symptoms may include trouble remembering where things were placed, failure to complete tasks, difficulty sustaining attention to nonengaging material, trouble sitting still during conversations, and frequently interrupting in social or work situations. In addition, ADHD is a heterogeneous condition that impacts various individuals differently in terms of symptom expression and functional impairment. Therefore, assessment of ADHD can present many challenges for the clinician who is frequently tasked with conducting an evaluation that requires differentiating from a multitude of disorders or even identifying a number of comorbidities. Clinicians should pay particular attention to the frequency and severity of the adult's behaviors and the extent to which the behaviors interfere with components of the individual's life such as friendships, occupational performance, home life, and community activities. Clinicians also may encounter clients that present at the initial appointment with a previous diagnosis of ADHD from another practitioner or with some form of past documentation of ADHD. Because the manifestation of ADHD can evolve over time and change depending on environmental context, it is recommended that clinicians conduct their own comprehensive assessment that evaluates for the presence or absence of current symptoms and associated level of impairment (Sibley et al., 2018).

**Many adults self-refer for an ADHD evaluation**

**Assessment and diagnosis of ADHD among adults is challenging because of comorbid conditions**

## 3.1 Assessment Procedures

**Obtaining collateral information is important for the assessment process**

When conducting a comprehensive evaluation to determine whether an adult meets criteria for a diagnosis of ADHD, it is recommended that practitioners obtain as much collateral information as available from other people who know the client well, such as a partner, spouse, or caregiver. According to the *DSM-5*, to qualify for an ADHD diagnosis during adulthood, there must be a history of several hyperactive-impulsive or inattentive symptoms (prior to 12 years of age) during childhood. These criteria allow for the possibility of an individual reporting several symptoms of ADHD but no associated impairment during childhood to then meet diagnostic criteria for ADHD later in life.

Multimethod assessment of ADHD in an adult should include the following components: (1) a thorough developmental history that includes a focus on social, behavioral, and medical history; (2) clinical interviews with the client and if possible the client's partner or parents; (3) rating scales or checklists completed by multiple informants for the purpose of capturing a broad perspective with regard to behaviors that may be associated with ADHD across settings (home, work, other activities); and (4) an evaluation of comorbid psychiatric diagnoses or learning disabilities.

Other assessment procedures that are more time intensive but may prove helpful in the diagnostic process include home or community observations and psychoeducational or neuropsychological testing for the purpose of assessing learning disabilities. Direct observations of the client's behavior in the home or recreational settings can be useful because they provide a way for the clinician to gain information about symptom expression in naturalistic contexts. Moreover, they capture an array of behaviors that a single office visit may not reveal. Although this information clearly can be informative to the diagnostic process, many mental health professionals who work with adult clients do not find this activity to be feasible because of the significant time requirement and lack of reimbursement. While psychoeducational or neuropsychological testing does not identify ADHD, these assessments can be useful for identifying other cognitive comorbidities such as specific learning disorders. The tools discussed in the following sections do not represent an exhaustive list of all available ADHD assessment techniques: Instead, these sections examine critical components of an ADHD evaluation and highlight corresponding evidence-based assessment strategies. For a more thorough discussion of the assessment of adult ADHD, see Lovett and Harrison (2021).

### 3.1.1 General Considerations

**Spouses, family members, or close friends may have different viewpoints regarding ADHD symptoms**

The diagnostic process ultimately must include assessing whether or not the adult meets criteria according to *DSM-5-TR* or *ICD-10* diagnostic criteria. There are several important issues for clinicians to consider prior to conducting an evaluation of an adult suspected of having ADHD. First, some adults with ADHD, like their younger counterparts, may have limited awareness of their difficulties and the resulting impairment and therefore may even underreport their behaviors. Second, different informants may provide different information and thus the various informants whom the clinician may interview are not in agreement and may bring their own biases to the assessment setting. For example, spouses may complain that their partner is disorganized and has trouble completing tasks: Alternatively, information from the caregivers may indicate that these behaviors were not present in childhood. Third, the symptom expression of ADHD may be variable and dependent on the situation or setting and context. For instance, adults may experience significant performance challenges if their job requires them to sit through long meetings and complete tasks on a tight schedule. Yet, these same individuals may fare well in a less structured home environment that does not require the completion of many organizational demands. Finally, clinicians should carefully assess whether an individual may be misrepresenting having symptoms of ADHD for the purpose of obtaining stimulant medication (Benson et al., 2015). "Faking to look bad" is a challenging endeavor in clinical practice given that there is no single test to confirm, or disconfirm, the diagnosis of ADHD. Adult populations that may be at higher risk of misusing or abusing stimulant medication include substance abusers, forensic populations, and adults that work in highly competitive vocations (Surman, 2013). Research suggests that over half of college students with a prescription for a stimulant were identified as likely malingering or overreporting their ADHD symptoms (Ramachandran et al., 2020).

### 3.1.2 Developmental History

Information about the client's developmental history can be gained through a structured or semistructured interview or through the use of a questionnaire administered to the client or the client's caregivers or partner/spouse. Information that is gathered for the developmental history usually focuses on the following domains: prenatal and perinatal history, developmental milestones, medical history, family history, treatment history, past and current (if applicable) school functioning, past and current social relationships, current behavioral concerns, and other concerns. To best utilize this information in the diagnostic process, clinicians should understand typical attentional development, emotional regulation, and age-appropriate behaviors and social skills. It also is important to note that an unremarkable developmental history does not automatically signify the absence of ADHD; rather a history significant for attentional problems likely suggests the presence of the disorder. Understanding the type of school and support system provided to the adult as a child and adolescent, and how they would have functioned without these, may uncover ADHD symptoms that may not have been apparent. For example, if the individual's parents consistently assisted with assignment completion, it may not have had an impact on their academic performance from the ADHD symptoms as a child. However, understanding if the adult's performance would have been impacted without these supports, or if there were impairment or distress related to implementation of these supports, can

**History can be obtained through interview or questionnaires completed by the client's partner**

clarify if there were childhood symptoms of ADHD. When childhood symptoms cannot be identified, examining temporal stability of symptoms, and ruling out alternative medical and psychiatric diagnostic explanations can help inform if symptoms are likely due to ADHD (Sibley, 2021).

### 3.1.3 Clinical Interview

**Clinical interviews are a mainstay of ADHD diagnosis**

The clinical interview is the foundation of a comprehensive ADHD assessment for evaluating both children and adults. However, there are several potential differences in the diagnostic process of ADHD among adults as compared to children. For example, when diagnosing ADHD among children, best practices suggest that data should be collected from multiple informants (e.g., child, caregivers, and teachers) to ensure that the child displays symptoms of ADHD that result in functional impairment across multiple domains (Barkley, 2015). However, this same standard of collecting data from multiple informants may be particularly challenging and arduous when assessing adults for ADHD. In part, this is due to the retrospective nature of the interview. In addition, caregivers of adults suspected of having ADHD may be unavailable and, when available, the clinician must carefully consider their ability to accurately recall onset and severity of ADHD symptoms (Kooij et al., 2010). There is some evidence to suggest that caregivers of adults with ADHD tend to overestimate age of symptom onset by approximately 5 years, even when health care records document an earlier age of onset. Attempts to corroborate symptom onset or severity with former teachers also may prove to be problematic. For example, primarily inattentive symptoms in childhood may not have been noticed in the classroom, and it may be challenging for teachers even if they can be found to accurately recall a student's classroom behavior that occurred many years in the past (Kooij et al., 2010). Research suggests that adults with chronic ADHD may underreport their symptoms compared to informant ratings (Sibley et al., 2016). Therefore, obtaining collateral information from the client's employer or spouse can be valuable if there is reported impairment in the work or home setting. However, clinicians must carefully consider privacy issues as there may be consequences if employers learn that their employee is suspected of having a diagnosis of ADHD.

Given the challenges associated with collecting information about childhood functioning from outside sources, the clinician may therefore choose to focus on corroborating current symptoms with individuals who are familiar with the client's symptoms in adulthood. Caregivers, spouses, partners, coworkers, and close friends can be crucial in assessing ADHD in an adult because they can provide a unique perspective on impairment across multiple settings. Caregivers are more accurate reporters of functional impairment than an adult with ADHD, and caregivers also may be better at reporting inattentive symptoms (Asherson et al., 2012). In addition, like children, adults with ADHD may have limited insight, inaccurate recall of symptoms or their severity, and struggle to correctly report the timing of onset of symptoms (Kooij et al., 2010). On the other hand, clinicians need to consider that spouses, partners, and close friends may not be aware of the extent of the client's difficulties, and clients often do not want employers or coworkers involved in the diagnostic process due to issues with stigma and privacy concerns (Lebowitz, 2013).

Clinicians also should seek to obtain any educational, psychological, and medical records that may elucidate the client's symptoms during childhood. When teacher interviews are not possible, the clinician may attempt to obtain important documentation for the diagnostic process such as school reports (Lovett & Harrison, 2021). Teachers' comments on report cards often include information regarding a child's academic difficulties or class behavior that may provide helpful insight into the client's early school experiences. Clinicians also may want to request records from any mental health treatment the client received during childhood to evaluate for potential comorbid disorders. For example, adults with symptoms of hyperactivity may have been referred for the management of conduct problems. In some cases, records from these professional contacts may be more informative than an interview with a provider who treated the child many years in the past.

**Clinicians should seek information from multiple sources when evaluating an individual for ADHD**

When conducting collateral interviews, the clinician must use clinical judgment to integrate observer reports into a clear picture of a client's clinical course. Unfortunately, it may not always be feasible to collect corroborating information from outside sources. Concerns about the practice of exclusively relying on self-report data include the phenomenon of "ADHD wannabes," a term referring to individuals who have self-diagnosed ADHD and present to the clinician seeking a formal diagnosis and/or medication (Barkley et al., 2008). In fact, clinicians who rely on self-report alone more commonly fail to diagnose ADHD when criteria are actually met (Kooij et al., 2010), potentially due to underreporting of symptoms (Sibley et al., 2016). Therefore, the astute clinician must use clinical judgment to ensure that adults unable to provide independent corroboration of symptoms still receive a thorough diagnostic evaluation. Due to the challenges in capturing the full picture of an adult's ADHD symptoms, Sibley (2021) recommends utilizing an "or rule," whereby one individual's report of symptom presence is sufficient to mark that symptom as present.

Clinicians can maximize their ability to obtain comprehensive and valid data by using a structured clinical interview designed specifically for assessing ADHD symptoms. Information should be collected regarding all *DSM-5* criteria for ADHD including: (1) frequency, severity, and persistence of symptoms; (2) age of onset and course of the disorder; (3) pervasiveness of symptoms across settings and situations; (4) functional impairments related to symptoms; and (5) potential comorbid diagnoses. Multiple clinical interviews using *DSM-5* criteria for ADHD in adults have been published. Clinical interviews using *DSM-IV* criteria can also be used with the understanding that the client needs to report only several symptoms with onset occurring before age 12 years.

The DIVA-5 (https://www.divacenter.eu/) is a recently published adult ADHD interview for *DSM-5* that assesses presence of ADHD symptoms in both adulthood and childhood concurrently by providing a question prompt and then examples of symptom presentation. The *DSM-IV* and *DSM-5* versions of the scale have been validated in a variety of languages (Hong et al., 2020; Ramos-Quiroga et al., 2019).

The ACE+ (https://www.psychology-services.uk.com/adhd) is a new clinical interview that was designed for *DSM-5* criteria for ADHD. Data on the reliability and validity of the measure have yet to be published. Like the DIVA-5, the ACE+ scale provides a prompt question and examples of symptom presentation in childhood and adulthood. The ACE+ enquires about each symptom presentation separately in home and occupational/academic settings with impairment only measured at the symptom level.

The Adult ADHD Clinical Diagnostic Scale (ACDS) v.1.2 is a semistructured interview widely used in adult ADHD research (Adler et al., 2015). The measure is distinct from those described above in that childhood ADHD is assessed separately from adult ADHD and symptom severity can be rated as part of the clinical interview.

The Conners' Adult ADHD Diagnostic Interview for DSM-IV (CAA-DID; Epstein et al., 2001) is comprehensive, easy to administer, and has demonstrated reliability and validity in diagnosing ADHD in adults (Epstein & Kollins, 2006). The first section of the CAA-DID, typically completed by the client, is designed to collect information regarding ADHD risk factors, developmental course, demographic history, and a screen for comorbid psychopathology. Given the strong heritability index for ADHD, demographic data regarding familial history of ADHD is relevant to the diagnostic process. Moreover, the relatively recent recognition of adult ADHD as a valid disorder means that the clinician should also collect information regarding cases of suspected ADHD among family members. The second portion of the CAA-DID consists of a clinical interview that systematically assesses *DSM-IV* criteria for ADHD. However, it is important to note that the CAA-DID does not adequately address item (E) of the *DSM-IV* or *DSM-5* ADHD criteria (see Section 1.2.1), which states that symptoms must not be better explained by another mental health disorder.

Structured interviews also can be used to comprehensively assess other psychiatric conditions that may partially or fully account for an individual's ADHD symptoms. A structured psychiatric interview that is commonly used in clinical practice is the Semi-Structured Clinical Interview for DSM-5 (SCID-5), which assesses mood, psychotic symptoms, anxiety, substance abuse, somatoform, eating, and adjustment disorders (First et al., 2016). Including the SCID in a diagnostic assessment for ADHD enables the clinician to ensure that an individual's symptoms of inattention, executive dysfunction, or impulsivity are not attributable to another psychiatric disorder (e.g., depression, schizophrenia). Results from the SCID also can provide guidance for treatment planning.

### 3.1.4 Behavioral Rating Scales

*Behavioral rating scales are a key element of the assessment of ADHD among adults*

Behavioral rating scales are crucial elements of evidence-based assessment of ADHD among adults. These instruments provide the clinician with a relatively quick and easily administered means of quantifying an individual's level of impairment relative to the normative population. Several rating scales have been developed for use with adults with suspected ADHD. It is important for clinicians to be aware that the results from a rating scale should not serve as the sole means of diagnosing ADHD in adults (Lovett & Harrison, 2021).

Among the most valid and reliable of the adult rating scales for ADHD is the Conners' Adult ADHD Rating Scales (CAARS; Conners et al., 1999), which are available in three different lengths (screening, short, and long versions). The CAARS instruments are organized into eight domains: inattentive/cognitive problems, hyperactivity/restlessness, impulsiveness/emotional lability, problems with self-concept, *DSM-IV* inattentive symptoms, *DSM-IV* hyperactive-impulsive symptoms, symptoms total, and an ADHD index. An inconsistency index is provided to assist the clinician in assessing the accuracy of reporting by the informant. T-scores are derived for each index, and the CAARS has a classification rate of 85% (Conners et al., 1999). A similar version of this instrument, the CAARS-O, can be used to obtain observer ratings of impairments from caregivers, spouses, or coworkers.

Another empirically based self-report rating scale for adult ADHD is the BAARS-IV (Barkley, 2011), which also conforms to *DSM-IV* diagnostic criteria. The BAARS-IV is available in quick- and long-screen forms, both of which can be completed in less than 7 minutes by the informant. The BAARS-IV assesses current and past childhood symptoms of ADHD and is cost-effective since the clinician can photocopy the instrument once it has been purchased. Like the CAARS instruments, the BAARS-IV features a self-report version and other-informant-report version that can be completed by an individual close to the client who is familiar with their functioning (e.g., a caregiver, partner, or spouse).

The ASRS is an 18-item symptom checklist structured on *DSM-IV/DSM-5* ADHD symptoms (Adler et al., 2013; Silverstein et al., 2018). Clinicians using the ASRS expanded version can also track symptoms commonly associated with ADHD (e.g., executive functioning, emotion regulation). The ASRS is publicly available, and a shorter version of the scale can be used to screen for adult ADHD (Kessler et al., 2005). Other psychometrically sound rating scales used in clinical practice include the ADHD Rating Scale 5 (DuPaul et al., 2016) and the Brown Attention-Deficit Disorder Scale (BADDS; Brown, 1996). It should be noted that the BADDS was developed prior to release of *DSM-IV* diagnostic criteria and therefore does not address the domain of hyperactivity and/or impulsivity. However, this scale is still widely used in clinical and research settings because of the prominence of inattentive symptoms in adult ADHD.

## 3.1.5 Differential Diagnosis/Comorbidities

Comorbid psychiatric diagnoses are prevalent in the adult ADHD population with some reports indicating that as many as 80% of adults with ADHD meet criteria for at least one additional diagnosis, the most common of which are

**Practitioners should assess for comorbid conditions when conducting an ADHD assessment**

mood, anxiety, and substance abuse disorders (Kooij et al., 2010). Because each of these disorders includes symptom areas of diagnostic overlap with ADHD, differential diagnosis can be challenging. However, accurate differential diagnosis and a thorough assessment of potential comorbid conditions are of paramount importance in the assessment of ADHD in adults. Therefore, it is recommended that broad-based structured clinical interviews (e.g., the SCID) be administered in combination with ADHD-specific measures to ensure comprehensive assessment of potential comorbidities.

### 3.1.6 Testing

To date, no neuropsychological tests provide sufficient sensitivity or specificity to diagnose ADHD independently (Holst & Thorell, 2016; Nikolas et al., 2019). Moreover, given the neurocognitive heterogeneity of ADHD, experts disagree as to the value of cognitive assessments in the diagnostic process (Barkley, 2019; Mapou, 2019). For example, although individuals with ADHD have consistently demonstrated lower full-scale IQ scores relative to those without the disorder (roughly .61 *SD* below the mean; Theiling & Petermann, 2016), the full-scale IQ cannot reliably be used as an indicator of ADHD. Intellectual assessment with an instrument such as the Wechsler Adult Intelligence Scale, 4th edition (WAIS-IV; Wechsler, 2008) may be helpful in differential diagnosis of possible comorbid learning or memory disorders (e.g., specific learning disorders) that may better explain ADHD symptoms or elucidate cognitive weaknesses that may be impacting academic or occupational performance.

*Psychoeducational & neuropsychological testing can assist in differential diagnosis*

Because ADHD is associated with impairments in executive functioning, assessment of executive performance in adults with suspected ADHD represents an important part of the diagnostic process (Barkley et al., 2010). A number of assessments are available for the practitioner. For example, the Conners' CPT-3 (Conners & Staff, 2014) is a 12-minute "go/no-go" assessment, tapping sustained attention, vigilance, response style, target and nontarget detection, reaction time, response style and variability, and impulsivity. The CPT-3 also yields classification ratings based on overall performance and individual domains to compare performance to the normative population. Other instruments used to assess executive functioning deficits in adults include the Stroop Color–Word Test (Stroop, 1935; Trenerry et al., 1989), the Wisconsin Card Sorting Test (Berg, 1948), and the Delis–Kaplan Executive Function System (Delis et al., 2001). These assessments yield data relevant to higher-order cognitive functions such as mental flexibility, perseveration, formulation of abstract concepts, problem-solving behavior, and inhibition. Although adults with ADHD frequently evidence impairment on each of these executive functioning assessments, the clinician is cautioned that results frequently have been inconsistent (Halperin & Schulz, 2006). As such, performance in the normative range on any individual test of intellectual or executive functioning should not be taken as an indication that an individual does not meet criteria for ADHD (Kooij et al., 2010). Similarly, poor performance on such instruments is not conclusively indicative of a diagnosis of ADHD. Rather, these assessments should be employed as part of a comprehensive evaluation of ADHD.

The following steps constitute a sample comprehensive evaluation procedure for older adolescents and adults:

1. an overview of the presenting problems and associated chronology, sources of the referral, a history that includes developmental, medical, academic, and social components, and an evaluation of behaviors intended to compensate for ADHD-related difficulties;
2. an analysis of the ways that symptoms may impact school, work, and recreation activities, as well as personal relationships;
3. collateral interviews with caregivers or a significant other that include their perspectives on the individual's symptoms and their impact, and the developmental, medical, and social history of the person who may have ADHD;
4. a psychological evaluation that investigates the presence of personality disorders as well as the potential presence of intellectual and developmental disabilities;
5. self-report measures that include general psychological symptoms, such as the Minnesota Multiphasic Personality Inventory-2, the Symptom Checklist 90 – revised (Derogatis, 1975), the Beck Depression Inventory-II (Beck et al., 1996), and the Beck Anxiety Inventory (Beck & Steer, 1993), as well as ADHD self-report checklists, such as the BAARS or the ASRS;
6. a semistructured psychological interview, such as the Barkley clinical interview form or the Brown ADD scales, that evaluates whether the client meets *DSM* criteria for ADHD; and
7. an assessment of cognitive, neuropsychological, and academic functioning that includes the WAIS-IV (Wechsler, 2008), the Wechsler Memory Scale-III, academic skills (e.g., reading and mathematics), a continuous performance test such as the Conners' CPT-3, and a test of executive functions.

## 3.2 The Decision-Making Process

Clinicians should consider all the information gathered during the assessment process to determine whether consistent and compelling evidence exists to support a diagnosis of ADHD (see Figure 1). Information from clinical interviews, behavioral rating scales, intellectual or neuropsychological tests, and assessment of comorbid symptoms or disorders should be integrated into a comprehensive assessment of an individual's current level of functioning. As noted above, the clinician should be aware that the lack of corroboration from outside reporters and/or test results in the normative range on intellectual or neuropsychological assessments do not necessarily indicate the absence of problems. Similarly, any deviation from the norm on one individual test does not conclusively support the presence of ADHD. First, observers may fail to

*Subthreshold symptoms can still impact functioning across a range of areas*

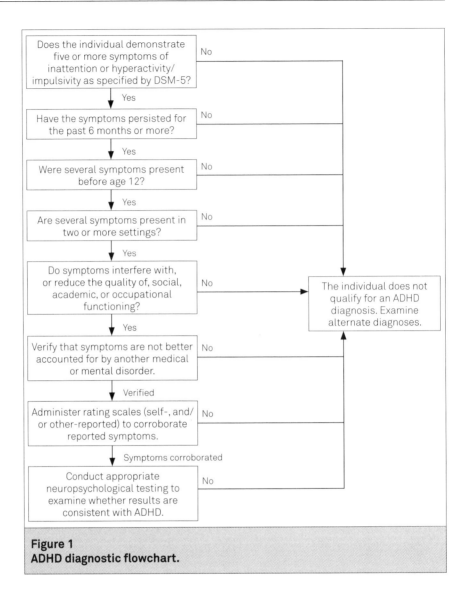

**Figure 1**
**ADHD diagnostic flowchart.**

corroborate clients' reports because many adults with ADHD try to minimize the degree to which others notice their symptoms (Holthe & Langvik, 2017). Therefore, it is possible that even a spouse or partner may be unaware of the extent of a client's difficulties. Second, ADHD is a heterogeneous condition in which adults may demonstrate deficits in some, but not all, areas of attention and executive functioning and overt symptoms of the disorder may be situation dependent (Barkley & Benton, 2021). For example, clinicians should be aware that the structure associated with testing environments likely does not reflect the actual settings in which adults suspected of ADHD need to perform on a daily basis. Testing is generally conducted in a quiet, one-on-one setting, in which the examinee has clear instructions and need only perform one structured task at a time. Thus, the environment does not ecologically reflect a natural setting in which an individual may normally need to demonstrate functional behaviors. Therefore, the provider must use astute clinical judgment to assess the level of executive impairment the client experiences outside the testing room. Finally, it should be noted that some individuals may fall short of meeting diagnostic criteria for the disorder by one or two symptoms, sometimes referred to as subthreshold disorder (i.e., where one of two symptoms are missing thereby failing to qualify an adult as meeting specific diagnostic criteria). This puts the practitioner in a dilemma since symptoms of ADHD also may require treatment, even though the symptoms are not all encompassing.

## 3.3   Treatment Considerations

Careful diagnostic interviewing and assessment is the gold standard of any case conceptualization and the formulation of treatment goals in the management of adults with ADHD. There are several unique factors in the management of ADHD among adults in comparison to children and adolescents. Caregivers typically manage treatment and adherence to therapy for children and adolescents, while this is not necessarily the case among adults. Some adult clients may live by themselves whereas for others the adult may sometimes rely on a significant other or family member for assistance with adherence to therapy including medication. Psychoeducation is important for adult clients regarding treatment modalities and specific aspects and components of treatment that may prove to be a formidable challenge for the client. An important aspect of assessment for the adult client is the specific aspect of treatment that may prove to be problematic for the client. Thus, social supports, strengths, and assets available to the patient with ADHD are important to assess. Specifically, family members or partners who are available to assist the client with various aspects of the treatment regimen will be important throughout the treatment process. In such cases, the client's family or spouse may be involved in assistance with treatment and as a result should be included as part of the treatment plan. Finally, while public awareness is growing at high pitch regarding ADHD among adults, as with many psychiatric disorders, there is a stigma associated with the disorder (Kooij et al., 2010), underscoring the need for ongoing supports and for psychoeducation with regard to the prevalence and symptoms associated with the disorder. The client must be informed that there exist efficacious treatments for ADHD and that this is a widespread disorder throughout the world thereby hopefully eliminating the stigma associated with the disorder.

Adults who receive a new diagnosis of ADHD are likely to be already involved in the mental health system due to the management of other psychiatric disorders or comorbidities relative to those who may have been identified with the disorder during childhood (Barkley et al., 2010; Evans et al., 2018). Thus, for adults suspected with ADHD, the astute practitioner should evaluate carefully for mood, anxiety, and substance use disorders. In addition to the presence of ADHD, a treatment plan also must be developed to address these aforementioned comorbidities. Such comorbidities can complicate the treatment of ADHD and increase the risk of suicidal ideation and impulsive behaviors among adults with ADHD (Barkley et al., 2010). The treatment and management of milder forms of anxiety and depression may be deferred at the commencement of treatment and, frequently, symptoms of these disorders may resolve independently when symptoms of ADHD are managed effectively (Kooij et al., 2010). Particularly if medication is warranted in managing ADHD, a close collaborative relationship should be formed with the individual's primary care provider or psychiatrist. The stimulants that are the most frequently employed pharmacotherapy to manage individuals with ADHD may exacerbate some specific comorbid mood disorders such as anxiety. Hence, the practitioner should inform the prescribing provider regarding the presence of these comorbid conditions. Finally, it should be noted that there is a high frequency of comorbidity of substance abuse disorders that occur among adults with ADHD and hence management of the substance abuse disorder including detoxification or rehabilitation may be initially indicated prior to the commencement of treatment for symptoms associated with ADHD (Chung & Bachrach, 2021).

Older adolescents or young adults with ADHD may frequently seek treatment in the context of their attending college or their employment setting. Thus, specific interventions within these domains may be warranted. Accommodations may be made in university settings as well as in employment settings under the Americans with Disabilities Act of 1990 (Weyandt & DuPaul, 2006), although the types of accommodation may vary by institutional setting. It may be more challenging to provide specific accommodations in the employment setting and, as a result, practitioners should familiarize themselves with the standards mandated by the Americans with Disabilities Act (see www.ada.gov) and when practitioners are in need of assistance in navigating clients within the system, referral to educational, vocational, or rehabilitation professionals may be necessary (Barkley et al., 2010).

Because older adolescents and young adults frequently experience challenges in the context of difficulties experienced in college or in the work setting, specific interventions or accommodations within these domains are frequently necessary. Appropriate documentations are often necessary for specific accommodations under the Americans With Disabilities Act, although the specific types of accommodation may differ in accordance with the institution or the program. Accommodations within the work setting may be variable and may depend on whether the employment is government related or is a private entity. In either case, the astute practitioner must familiarize themselves with those standards evidenced by the Americans with Disabilities Act. When the provider is not fully knowledgeable about how to assist clients in navigating the system, a referral to an educational, vocational, or rehabilitation professional may be warranted (Barkley et al., 2010).

# 4

# Treatment

## 4.1 Methods of Treatment

ADHD is a chronic neurodevelopmental disorder that is common in adults but also frequently underdiagnosed. Although the symptoms of ADHD begin in childhood, some individuals will not be diagnosed with ADHD until their adult years. For those individuals diagnosed with ADHD in childhood, some research suggests that 90% will retain at least some of the ADHD symptoms in adulthood although the course of the disorder and symptom presentation may fluctuate (Sibley et al., 2022). The chronic course of the disorder has several implications for treatment of ADHD among adults. First, clinicians should emphasize to affected individuals and their partners, spouses, or family members that ADHD in most cases results in a need for continual, coordinated care (Barkley & Benton, 2021). Second, the symptoms and problems associated with ADHD may vary and be expressed differently across the life span. For example, many adults report diminished levels of hyperactivity from childhood to adulthood, but still endorse restlessness or fidgetiness. Third, intervention is critical to help prevent and/or ameliorate the short- and long-term consequences of the disorder. Lastly, when implementing treatment plans, clinicians should take a long-term view. Even when treatment results in a reduction of the core symptoms of ADHD in the short term, there may still be persistent associated problems (e.g., social challenges) or functional impairments (e.g., occupational performance) that require continued intervention.

Although there is no cure for ADHD, there are well-established and evidence-based options for the treatment of adults with the disorder that include pharmacological interventions, CBT, supportive and family therapy, psychoeducational interventions, and combined treatments. Because of the heterogeneity of ADHD symptoms and needs among those with the disorder, it is likely that various treatment plans will be appropriate for different adults. In addition, research suggests that multimodal therapies work best for ADHD when the disorder is comorbid with other psychiatric disorders and that when ADHD coexists with other comorbid psychiatric conditions in adults, the most impairing condition should generally be treated first (Katzman et al., 2017). In some cases, the treatments may be more effective for the comorbid disorder than for the ADHD. When choosing a treatment plan, it is often helpful for affected individuals and their spouses, partners, or family members to pinpoint specific behaviors and challenges to address. Once

*Treatments for ADHD include pharmacological, psychosocial, psychoeducation, and combined treatments*

these goals are identified, it is easier to tailor compensatory strategies to the problem areas as well as assess whether specific interventions are effective.

### 4.1.1 Psychopharmacology

Compared to the substantial body of research conducted on pharmacotherapy for children with ADHD, far fewer controlled studies have examined medication therapy in adults. Nonetheless, because medications used to effectively treat children with ADHD also benefit adults with ADHD, some experts consider pharmacotherapy to be the primary treatment option for adults with ADHD (Mattingly et al., 2021). The most commonly prescribed psychotropic medications for the treatment of ADHD among adults is the class of agents known as stimulants. The prescribing and usage of stimulants – mostly for the treatment of ADHD – has increased dramatically. For example, total stimulant usage doubled in the years 2006–2016 (Piper et al., 2018). Due, in part, to increases in the use of medication to treat ADHD, controversy and public debate continue about whether stimulants are being overly prescribed for management of the disorder in young people and adults.

Many explanations have been suggested for the increase in prescriptions that include, but are not limited to, an increase in public and practitioner recognition and acceptance of ADHD as a real disorder, a broadening of the diagnostic criteria for ADHD in *DSM-5*, less stigma than in previous years for medication as a treatment option, a recognition that there are specific subgroups of the disorder, an increase in the availability of specialized services for assessing and treating ADHD, and the use of stimulants to treat other disorders such as obesity and narcolepsy (Piper et al., 2018).

Before discussing specific stimulant medications with adults with ADHD, it is important to address the affected individual's understanding and expectations regarding stimulants and their effects, and to provide psychoeducation about the benefits as well as the potential adverse side effects of these medications. With some of the newer stimulants (e.g., medications that are longer acting and therefore require fewer doses), research has generally suggested that approximately 70% of adults respond to the stimulants (Advokat & Scheithauer, 2013). Stimulant medications have been demonstrated to improve some of the specific core cognitive and behavioral symptoms associated with ADHD in the short term. Stimulants are effective in enhancing attention and concentration while also reducing impulsivity and fidgetiness for adults with ADHD (Advokat & Scheithauer, 2013).

Individuals should be informed that there are also some major limitations of stimulant treatment. There are individual differences in response to medication, and not all adults will positively respond to these medications (Piper et al., 2018). And, for those adults who demonstrate a positive response, this rarely equates with a normalizing of their behavior. Interestingly, the stimulants have limited impact on domains of functional impairment associated with ADHD, including problems with social behavior, organization, time management, and prioritizing, which are frequently the primary reason that adults seek treatment. Another significant limitation is that no long-term effects have been established for stimulant medication. Other classes of psychotropics (e.g., specific serotonin reuptake inhibitors) may prove more effective for ADHD when it is comorbid with anxiety disorder or depression. Finally, the stimulants may be contraindicated for adults who are actively abusing substances or who have a spouse or partner with a substance abuse disorder.

Approximately 75% of adults with ADHD have at least one comorbid condition. Practitioners should be aware that some symptoms associated with comorbid disorders may negatively impact response to medication for adults with ADHD (Piper et al., 2018). In general, conditions that are considered more severe should be treated first. Following improvement with the more impairing disorder, the other condition can then be treated. For example, if depression is considered the more impairing condition, practitioners should initiate treatment (e.g., antidepressant medication, CBT) that focuses on ameliorating the depressive symptoms prior to treating ADHD. In the case of an adult presenting with co-occurring ADHD and a substance use disorder, the focus of treatment should be on addressing the substance use problem (Piper et al., 2018). This is especially important given that the use of stimulants is contraindicated for adults actively abusing substances.

*Stimulant medications are contraindicated for adults actively abusing substances*

There is no evidence to suggest that stimulant use increases the chance of an individual developing problems with substance use or dependence. In fact, several meta-analyses found that the use of stimulant medication during childhood either reduced or did not increase the risk for substance abuse in adulthood (Humphreys et al., 2013; Schoenfelder et al., 2014). Because the stimulants have significant abuse potential, adults with ADHD should be assessed for substance abuse or diversion before being prescribed a stimulant medication. If the adult is abusing or suspected of abusing drugs, prescribing a nonstimulant medication for ADHD is recommended. Clinicians should actively monitor the response to medication in all adults and should proceed with special care in the case of dual diagnoses, particularly substance abuse. The risk of abuse is lower for the longer-acting stimulants (e.g., Concerta, Adderall XR, Vyvanse) relative to the short-acting stimulants that can be inhaled (e.g., Ritalin, Adderall, Dexedrine).

There are no explicit guidelines to help determine which stimulant medication to use first when treating an adult with ADHD although some experts suggest amphetamine-based medication over methylphenidate as the first-choice stimulant for adults (Cortese et al., 2018). It is more common in clinical practice for prescribers to use long-acting formulations instead of short-acting medications. Individuals with ADHD who do not observe benefits from one stimulant medication will often respond to another (Piper et al., 2018), and response to one stimulant does not predict response to others. A meta-analysis yielded relatively similar effect sizes for immediate-release (0.96) and long-acting (0.73) stimulants for the treatment of ADHD in adults, both of which were greater relative to the effect sizes for nonstimulant medications for the management of the ADHD disorder (Faraone & Glatt, 2009).

**Use of stimulant medication must be carefully monitored for side effects**

All medication effects must be carefully monitored by clinicians. Treatment-emergent adverse side effects from stimulant medication may include decreased appetite, stomachache, insomnia, and headache (Piper et al., 2018). Less common side effects include motor tics, headaches, nausea, fatigue, irritability, and increases in heart rate and blood pressure. Many side effects associated with the stimulants abate after a short period, or may disappear if the dosage or timing of administration is adjusted (Piper et al., 2018).

### 4.1.2 Stimulant Medications

**Methylphenidate-based and amphetamine/ dextroamphetamine-based medications are approved by the FDA**

There are two groups of stimulant medications frequently prescribed for the treatment of ADHD among adults, each based on a different stimulant compound: methylphenidate-based medications and amphetamine/dextroamphetamine-based medications. These compounds are considered Schedule II drugs because of the potential for abuse when not used as medically prescribed. Therefore, psychostimulants are regulated by the Drug Enforcement Administration.

There are short-acting (Ritalin, Methylin, Focalin), intermediate (Ritalin SR, Methylin ER, Metadate ER, Metadate CD, Ritalin LA), and long-acting versions of methylphenidate (Concerta, Focalin XR, Daytrana patch, Quillivant XR). Similarly, there are short-acting (Dexedrine, Dextrostat), intermediate (Adderall, Dexedrine spansules), and long-acting formulas of amphetamine/dextroamphetamine (Adderall XR, Vyvanse). Brief descriptions of some of these specific drugs are in Table 2.

The short-acting formula of methylphenidate (e.g., Ritalin, Methylin) is often administered twice a day, usually in the morning and early afternoon. The recommended starting dose of immediate-release methylphenidate is 5 mg, increasing in 5 mg increments up to 20 mg per dose. Ritalin can be consumed in 5 mg, 10 mg, or 20 mg tablets. Though the average dosage is 20–30 mg daily, there are adults who may need 40–60 mg, and others who will demonstrate symptom improvement on just 10–15 mg daily. Because immediate release methylphenidate is fast acting, the medication usually begins working about 15–30 minutes after ingestion, with beneficial effects being observed after 30–60 minutes, and peak effect occurring on average 90–120 minutes after it is taken, although this is frequently variable. For short-acting preparations, the effects can last from 2 to 4 hours. Although two doses per day is typical, the prescribing physician may decide in some cases that a third dose after work is warranted if the adult continues to experience significant difficulties in the evening or experiences a rebound effect. Because stimulants can wear off rapidly and leave the brain receptors too quickly, there may be a rebound effect whereby the adult demonstrates increased irritability, emotional lability, and an exacerbation of the core symptoms of ADHD (Kolar et al., 2008). The third dose of medication is usually half of the normal dose and is given about 30 minutes before the expected rebound symptoms for the purpose of easing the dissipation of the medication.

## Table 2
### FDA-Approved Medications for the Management of ADHD Symptoms

| Type | Class | Brand name | Form Short-acting | Form Long-acting | Common side effects |
|---|---|---|---|---|---|
| **Stimulant medications** | Amphetamine | Adderall | ✓ | | Loss of appetite, weight loss, sleep difficulties, irritability, tics |
| | | Adderall XR | | ✓ | |
| | | Adzenys ER | | ✓ | |
| | | Adzenys XR-ODT | | ✓ | |
| | | Desoxyn | | ✓ | |
| | | Dexedrine | Intermediate | | |
| | | Dyanavel XR | | ✓ | |
| | | Evekeo | ✓ | | |
| | | Evekeo ODT | ✓ | | |
| | | Mydayis | | ✓ | |
| | | ProCentra | ✓ | | |
| | | Vyvanse chewable | | ✓ | |
| | | Vyvanse capsule | | ✓ | |
| | | Zenzedi | ✓ | | |
| | Methylphenidate | Adhansia XR | | ✓ | |
| | | Azstarys | | ✓ | |
| | | Aptensio XR | Intermediate | | |
| | | Concerta | | ✓ | |
| | | Cotempla XR-ODT | | ✓ | |
| | | Daytrana patch | | ✓ | |
| | | Focalin | ✓ | | |
| | | Focalin XR | | ✓ | |
| | | Jornay PM | | ✓ | |
| | | Metadate CD | Intermediate | | |
| | | Metadate ER | | ✓ | |
| | | Methylin chewable | ✓ | | |
| | | Methylin ER | Intermediate | | |

### Table 2 continued

| Type | Class | Brand name | Form Short-acting | Form Long-acting | Common side effects |
|---|---|---|---|---|---|
| | | Methylin oral solution | ✓ | | |
| | | QuilliChew ER | | ✓ | |
| | | Quillivant XR | | ✓ | |
| | | Ritalin | ✓ | | |
| | | Ritalin LA | Intermediate | | |
| | | Ritalin SR | Intermediate | | |
| Nonstimulant medications | Norepinephrine reuptake inhibitor | Qelbree | | ✓ | Sleep difficulties, anxiety, fatigue, upset stomach, dizziness, dry mouth |
| | | Strattera | | ✓ | |
| | Alpha agonist | Intuniv | | ✓ | Sleepiness, headache, fatigue, abdominal pain |
| | | Kapvay | | ✓ | |

The intermediate-acting extended release tablets are usually taken once or twice a day. Ritalin SR is a sustained release preparation tablet that initially releases 10 mg of methylphenidate, followed by an additional 10 mg approximately 4 hours later for a total duration of action of 8 hours. Since individuals metabolize medications differently, some adults will derive greater benefit from two tablets, 4 hours apart, than one timed-release administration. The long-acting formulas are usually taken once a day and effects can last from 8 to 12 hours. Concerta is a long-acting form of methylphenidate, and is available in 18 mg, 27 mg, 36 mg, and 54 mg tablets. It uses a time-released system by means of an osmotic pump within the capsule to regulate consistent release of the medication throughout the course of the day. Another methylphenidate preparation, Metadate CD, delivers 30% of the dose immediately, and continually releases the remainder of the medication throughout the day.

Dextroamphetamine is prepared in several different ways. The short-acting version (Dexedrine) is in tablet form of 5 mg and 10 mg and on average one to three tablets are provided for each dose every 4 to 5 hours. Dexedrine spansules are available in 5 mg, 10 mg, and 15 mg, and usually have an effect that lasts for about 6 to 8 hours. Dexedrine spansules may take up to 1 hour to be effective. Other variants of dextroamphetamine include amphetamine salt tablets (Adderall) that usually last about 6 hours and are given once or twice a day depending on the length of therapeutic effect. Adderall XR is the longer-acting amphetamine preparation and provides control of ADHD symptoms for up to 12 hours. Vyvanse is considered a prodrug because it is inactive until metabolized in the body. The mechanism of action is thought to help prevent abuse of the drug that has been found to occur with Adderall.

Several stimulant preparations have been developed for those cases in which the oral forms are not well tolerated, when the adult has difficulty with pill swallowing, or when there are issues of compliance. Daytrana is a methylphenidate patch that can be used as an alternative to orally administered medications. The patch is attached to the individual's skin near the hip and can be worn for up to 9 hours daily. For adults who have trouble swallowing pills, Focalin is a stimulant that comes in a capsule, and can be opened and sprinkled on foods.

Other ADHD stimulant medications recently introduced and approved by the Food and Drug Administration (FDA) in 2019 for use with adults with ADHD include Jornay PM and Adhansia XR. Different from other stimulant mediations, Jornay PM is taken in the evening so that the medication begins working by the time the patient wakes and through the rest of the day. Adhansia XR is available in six extended-release capsules, which include some of the highest dosage strengths currently on the market.

Adults generally respond to stimulants in a dose-related manner (Stevens et al., 2013). However, because individual responses to stimulant medication can be variable, health professionals should collaborate with the adult with ADHD to carefully evaluate their response to medication. Stimulants should be carefully and gradually titrated so that an optimal dose is reached, i.e., one that manages specific target behaviors (e.g., inattention) while still resulting in the fewest adverse side effects. The dose is at an appropriate level when maximum benefits can be observed, and adverse side effects are at a minimum. Some evidence indicates that underdosing results in decreased effectiveness (Farhat et al., 2022). During the titration period, the medication should be used for 7 days, so that changes can be observed across a range of settings. During this period, the affected adult and their spouse, partner, or other family members should attempt to observe the effects of medication over the course of each day and compare these observations with the structure of environmental demands. It is especially useful to note the times of day when the effects of medication begin to dissipate, and to attempt to have these times correspond to recreation or mealtimes or other situations where high levels of concentration are not required. In addition, ingesting stimulants with meals or snacks can help alleviate some common adverse side effects, such as gastrointestinal inflammation.

*Adults' response to medication should be carefully monitored*

### 4.1.3 Nonstimulant Medications

Atomoxetine (Strattera) is a nonstimulant medication approved by the FDA in 2002 for the treatment of ADHD in children, adolescents, and adults. It is in a class of drugs called norepinephrine reuptake inhibitors because it affects the transmitters of norepinephrine, a natural substance in the brain that helps manage behavior. Atomoxetine is not classified as a stimulant, although it does have some stimulant effects. It is not a drug that

*Several nonstimulant medications have been approved by the FDA for the treatment of ADHD*

is abused by users, and prescriptions for the drug can be written without Schedule II restrictions because it is not classified as a stimulant medication. Atomoxetine is usually taken either once or twice daily. It lasts for 24 hours and therefore provides a therapeutic effect that lasts throughout the day and night. In contrast to the stimulants, dosing for atomoxetine is based on weight and full therapeutic effect may not be achieved until the adult has taken it for 3–4 weeks.

Another psychotropic therapy for ADHD is Modafinil (Provigil), which is a cognitive-enhancement agent primarily used to promote wakefulness. Modafinil differs structurally from other drugs for ADHD, and selectively targets the cerebral cortex (Elliott et al., 2020). It has been prescribed as an off-label treatment for ADHD. Modafinil is usually administered once daily, with dosage levels of approximately 170–425 mg. Qelbree is the most recent nonstimulant approved for the treatment of ADHD in adults.

Clonidine (Catapres, Nexicon) and guanfacine (Tenex) are alpha-adrenergic agonists that also come in long-acting 24-hour-release versions (Kapvay and Intuniv). Because these medicines have proven most effective in reducing hyperactive and aggressive behaviors in children, their use in adults has generally been minimal.

For adults with comorbid diagnoses, particularly comorbidity of the internalizing disorders (e.g., anxiety disorders or depression), other psychotropic medications that target depression, anxiety, or mood lability may be prescribed. Notably, none of the antidepressants has been approved by the FDA for the management of ADHD in adults and therefore treatment of symptoms related to ADHD would be considered off label (Verbeeck et al., 2017). Adults may be prescribed tricyclic antidepressants, including Imipramine (Tofranil), Nortryptaline (Pamelor) and Desipramine (Norpramine). Other physicians prescribe bupropion (Wellbutrin) or venlafaxine (Effexor).

*Collaboration is important when making treatment decisions about medication*

For adults with ADHD, medication decisions should be reached through collaboration between the affected individual, their spouse, partner, or other family members, and medical personnel. Before an adult begins a medication regimen, they should undergo a physical evaluation to determine whether there are any preexisting medical conditions. When adults begin taking medications for ADHD, they should begin with a low dose of the drug (typically 5 mg for the immediate-release formulations; starting doses are more variable for the intermediate- and long-acting formulations), and gradually increase the dose. It is recommended that prescribing physicians monitor medication effects weekly during the titration period, and monthly once medication doses are established. Based on each adult's specific response to the medication, health professionals can determine the dose that is best suited to the adult for the specific target symptoms to be addressed. In the weeks and months following the commencement of drug treatment, adults should monitor and evaluate ADHD symptoms and adverse side effects in collaboration with family members and clinicians. Measures to assess the adult's response to medication should be like those assessments used to diagnose and identify specific target behaviors for which the medication may be intended.

## 4.1.4 Psychosocial and Psychological Therapies

The research related to psychosocial and psychological treatments for adults with ADHD is more limited than research related to pharmacological approaches for treating adult ADHD. Findings from a recent meta-analysis of the long-term efficacy of psychosocial treatments for adults with ADHD revealed that treatment groups evidenced greater improvement than control groups in self-reported total ADHD symptoms, inattention, and hyperactivity/impulsivity, and on a measure of global functioning, and these gains were generally maintained for at least 12 months (López-Pinar et al., 2018). The most employed and studied psychosocial and psychological therapies for adults with ADHD include coaching and CBT, metacognitive therapy (e.g., time-management and organizational-skills training), and supportive and family therapy. Also reviewed below are neurofeedback and cognitive-enhancement therapies (see Section 4.1.8) given their increasing use for treating ADHD among young people and adults. Finally, aspects of psychoeducation (Section 4.1.9), which should always be a component of ADHD treatment, are described.

> Psychosocial and psychological treatments may be useful for adults with ADHD

## 4.1.5 Coaching and CBT

Coaching and CBT, which can be delivered in individual and group formats, share many components in that both modalities seek to provide structure for the adult suffering with ADHD and focus on teaching coping and problem-solving skills for identified problems. When working with an adult with ADHD, the following coaching and CBT strategies may be used as part of a treatment plan: (1) helping the client to gain acceptance of the disorder; (2) strengthening their time-management skills; (3) setting realistic goals; (4) improving their organizational skills across settings; (5) addressing difficulties in interpersonal relationships; (6) develop behavioral goals for starting and completing tasks; and (7) helping clients to better understand the association between their emotional reactions and ADHD (Kooji et al., 2010). Strategies more directly associated with CBT include helping clients identify and modify negative cognitions associated with avoidance of tasks ("As usual, this is too hard to do"), lack of motivation (e.g., "I am too lazy"), and negative affect (e.g., "I am no good") (Safren et al., 2005). Therapists then assist the client in challenging these dysfunctional cognitions with the goal of diminishing hopelessness as well as improving motivation. A systematic review of psychosocial treatments of ADHD in adults concluded that CBT was the most effective treatment modality for reducing symptoms of ADHD as well as comorbid symptoms of anxiety and depression (Vidal-Estrada et al., 2012). A recent systematic review and meta-analysis indicated that the available evidence supports a recommendation for CBT for adults (Tourjman et al., 2022). For an in-depth review of CBTs for adults with ADHD, see Knouse (2015).

## 4.1.6 Metacognitive Therapy: Time-Management and Organizational-Skills Training

>  Practitioners should help adults develop more effective organization and time-management strategies

Many adults with ADHD struggle with personal and professional activities that require organization and management of time. For example, these individuals may have trouble paying their bills on time, their home and office space may be messy and cluttered, they may be chronically late for work or miss assignments and deadlines, and they may frequently misplace important objects (e.g., car keys). This general disorganization, in turn, has a negative impact on interpersonal relationships, occupational performance, financial stability, and their overall quality of life (Barkley & Benton, 2021). Although there is a compelling evidence base for medication for the treatment of the core symptoms of ADHD, there is little evidence to suggest that treatment with stimulant medication improves disorganization, poor time management, and procrastination (Langberg et al., 2008), which comprise the issues that frequently cause the most problems for many adults with ADHD. Therefore, practitioners working with adults with ADHD may be tasked with implementing skills and strategy training that focuses on helping clients develop more effective strategies to structure and organize their environment and improve their time management. Often, adults with ADHD struggle to balance the competing demands between their home and professional responsibilities. Thus, common target behaviors as part of this training include helping adults prioritize these responsibilities and complete tasks within an appropriate time frame (Langberg et al., 2008). Spouses, partners, and other loved ones also can influence success with organization by helping adults with ADHD to use brief to-do lists and planners, sit with them when balancing a checkbook, and setting specific times for reviewing financial records.

A metacognitive approach that utilizes cognitive-behavioral principles is the guiding framework for organizational interventions with adults. Practitioners work with their clients to challenge and ultimately reduce maladaptive cognitions while also replacing them with more accurate cognitions. For example, adults with ADHD may think, "there are too many bills to pay, and I am never going to get them all paid on time so I might as well give up." This statement can be challenged and reframed with a more realistic cognition, such as, "there are a lot of bills to pay, but if I set and to stick to a schedule, I will be able to get them all done within a reasonable time frame." For behavioral reinforcement, adults with ADHD can collaboratively partner with the practitioner to determine appropriate rewards for completing tasks (e.g., going out to dinner or buying a gift for themselves).

Most studies that investigated stand-alone organizational interventions for individuals with ADHD have focused on the child population; however, several studies have been conducted with adults. In a series of studies that used an 8-week and 12-week group intervention format, Solanto and colleagues (2008) focused on the following elements: (1) setting realistic goals; (2) effective use of a daily planner and organizer; (3) strategies for breaking down complex tasks; (4) strategies for accurate estimation of time; and

(5) dividing of physical space into "organizational zones." Results revealed that participants made significant pre- to posttreatment gains in self-reported symptoms of inattention and organization. There were no significant between group differences for the 8-week and 12-week versions. Notably, a limitation of this study was the lack of any control groups. In a follow-up study that used a randomized controlled design, Solanto and colleagues (2010) reported significantly greater improvements in severity of ADHD symptoms among individuals receiving metacognitive therapy as compared to individuals treated with supportive therapy.

### 4.1.7 Supportive and Family Therapies

Because many adults with ADHD also have other psychological symptoms that may include depression or anxiety, supportive and/or family therapy can address aspects of functioning that may not necessarily be responsive to pharmacotherapy. These therapy modalities also can target issues common to adults with ADHD, such as low self-esteem and self-efficacy, marital difficulties, and problems with anger management. Many adults with ADHD, especially those who have yet to receive intervention, have had to endure others' assessments of them as "lazy, ineffective, and unfocused." Others may have recognized the adult's functional deficits and attributed these impairments to inherent personality or temperamental characteristics rather than a neurodevelopmental disorder. Since adults affected by ADHD have often internalized these negative messages, thereby impacting self-esteem, psychological interventions can help target and correct these inaccurate judgments and their effects on self-schemas.

*Supportive and family therapies address low self esteem, relationship difficulties, and problems with anger management*

### 4.1.8 Neurofeedback and Cognitive-Enhancement Training

Neurofeedback training seeks to improve cognitive deficits in adults with ADHD by providing feedback from brain waves as measured by electroencephalography. Cognitive-enhancement training utilizing computers is a relatively new treatment modality for adults with ADHD. The computerized training targets improvements in working memory and attention through practice and immediate performance feedback (Sibley et al., 2014). The intervention takes the form of a software program that individuals use over the course of several weeks. There have been few randomized clinical trials conducted that systematically examined the effectiveness of neurofeedback training or cognitive-enhancement training in adults with ADHD. Therefore, given the lack of available evidence, practitioners should be cautious about the use of neurofeedback and cognitive-enhancement training to treat symptoms of ADHD among adults.

*Cognitive-enhancement training seeks to improve working memory and attention*

### 4.1.9 Psychoeducation

Regardless of whether the treatment plan focuses on medication management, time-management or organizational strategies, psychosocial/cognitive-behavioral intervention, or a combination of therapies, practitioners are encouraged to provide psychoeducation to the adult and their partner, spouses, or family members. Psychoeducational components often comprise a key element of success, and clients, partners, or family members may need to be trained in the most effective ways to advocate for those with ADHD. In addition to the use of psychotherapy or medication, many health care professionals may refer their clients to helpful books, videotapes, or internet sites that provide accessible information regarding the etiology and management of ADHD. A number of these sources are provided in the Appendix.

Some adults with ADHD or their partners or spouses may find it helpful to join self-help or support groups. CHADD (Children and Adults with Attention-Deficit Disorder) and the National Attention Deficit Disorder Association both provide information, support, and resources for individuals and families affected by ADHD. These groups are often helpful in providing current information about ADHD and offer the benefits of a support network that may assist individuals and their significant others to cope with the disorder and become effective advocates either for themselves or their family members.

## 4.2 Mechanisms of Action

There is a preponderance of evidence that there exist deficiencies in the reuptake of neurotransmitters at the level of the synapses, particularly for the neurotransmitters of dopamine and norepinephrine among those individuals with ADHD relative to their typical peers. Epinephrine and serotonin also have been implicated in the mechanisms associated with ADHD. It is hypothesized that the increase in neurotransmitter availability at the synapses leads to the enhancement of extracellular dopamine and norepinephrine activity in the central nervous system, particularly in the prefrontal cortex and basal ganglia regions of the brain. Stimulant medication increases neurotransmitter activity and inhibits problematic behavior associated with impulsivity, as well as enhancing attention, concentration, self-regulation, and executive functioning (for reviews, see Kapalka et al., 2018).

The various stimulants are posited to exert effects of neurochemical processes (Brown, in press). For example, one frequently employed stimulant, methylphenidate, is believed to block the dopamine transporter within the synaptic cleft, which in turn increases the release of dopamine. This process is believed to enhance attention, focus, and concentration among individuals who have impaired dopaminergic signals, a hypothesized deficit among individuals with ADHD. There is compelling evidence from functional neuroimaging studies including positron emission tomography techniques as well as investigations of brain connectivity to indicate that the stimulants potentiate and activate blood flow as well as electrical activity in the regions of the brain that is responsible for goal directed, task-oriented behavior, such as the executive function networks (for a review, see Barkley, 2022). Specifically, results from positron emission tomography studies have demonstrated that the therapeutic levels of methylphenidate block over one half of the brain's dopamine transporters and increase the concentration of dopamine in the basal ganglia (Volkow et al., 2002). Amphetamine, a stimulant similar to methylphenidate, is believed to exert its therapeutic effect by elevating extracellular dopamine; however, its action is that it prolongs dopamine receptor signaling in the striatum.

Mechanisms of action for the nonstimulants share some similarities and differences when compared to the stimulants. Tricyclic antidepressants are an alternative therapy for the management of ADHD but are only employed in rare circumstances and under careful supervision because they pose the risk of significant cardiac toxicity. Atomoxetine is a nonstimulant therapy approved by the FDA for managing ADHD in children and adolescents and had been considered a first alternative for those who do not respond to the stimulants. Atomoxetine is a selective inhibitor of the neurotransmitter norepinephrine. Atomoxetine is posited to inhibit presynaptic norepinephrine reuptake, thereby increasing extracellular norepinephrine and the increase in dopamine in the prefrontal cortex is thus more indirect (for a review, see Nigg & Barkley, 2014). Another class of medications used to manage ADHD are the alpha-adrenergic agonists, which may pose considerable cardiac risks, particularly because these agents were originally designed to decrease blood pressure and tachycardia. The FDA approved an extended-release form of one alpha-adrenergic, guanfacine, which has a very different mechanism of action than either the stimulants or atomoxetine. Guanfacine is believed to fine-tune the alpha-2 receptors on nerve cells in the prefrontal cortex thereby producing enhanced signal strength and conductivity (Nigg & Barkley, 2014). The therapeutic effects of the alpha-adrenergics on the prefrontal cortex have been demonstrated to enhance attention and other cognitive impairments associated with ADHD (for a review, see Kapalka et al., 2018).

Psychotherapy is likely to enhance functional outcomes for adults with ADHD in a number of ways. Specifically, structured forms of psychotherapy may assist individuals with ADHD in the formulation of goals, identifying obstacles to accomplishing such goals, and meeting those challenges in ways that may be applied to the challenges associated with daily living. In addition, psychoeducation for ADHD may enable adults and their partners as well as family members to ascertain an enhanced understanding of this lifelong disorder and ultimately assist them in making more informed treatment decisions. Finally, family systems psychotherapy can assist the entire family in meeting the demands associated with ADHD and particularly those symptoms of the disorder that might impact the entire family.

Behavioral approaches as well as cognitive-behavioral interventions have their origins in contingency management and social learning theory. The goal of such therapies is to offer adults and their significant others as well as family members specific tools and avenues with which they can address those behavioral difficulties they experience that are associated with ADHD. When the individual with ADHD and their loved ones, including the clinician, agree on those strategies necessary to incorporate for the purpose of coping with the disorder, these strategies may be practiced both within and outside of the therapy sessions. Such strategies might include list making, creating specific times set aside for the organization of tasks, and the assessment of plans and priorities. In this way adults with ADHD may learn new methods and ways of living that can replace old patterns and habits. Similarly, for spouses and partners whose relationship is apt to be significantly affected by ADHD, learning new and effective strategies for interacting with adults with ADHD will demand an initial investment of time and practice. When new methods are eventually learned, they may be internalized and become automatic thereby producing consistent and effective responses that mitigate undesirable behaviors and promulgate positive actions. Thus, changes in the interaction styles and the use of new strategies are conceptualized as the mechanism of action whereby CBT influences the behavior of adults with ADHD.

## 4.3  Efficacy and Prognosis

*Prognosis among different individuals with ADHD varies widely*

Although ADHD is considered a chronic disorder, prognosis among different individuals with ADHD may vary widely. It was previously thought that a sizable percentage of adults with ADHD could experience full remission of symptoms and therefore would not meet *DSM* criteria. However, the available literature from the MTA study revealed that most participants with ADHD (63.8%) had fluctuating periods of remission and recurrence over the period of childhood to young adulthood (Sibley et al., 2022). Thus, the authors highlighted that most individuals with ADHD will experience waxing and waning of their symptoms with periods of full remission that are more often temporary than sustained. Most experts agree that ADHD symptoms that persist into adulthood are associated with considerable functional impairments. For example, adults with ADHD evidence worse outcomes in educational, occupational, social, and family domains as compared to adults with no history of the disorder (Kooij et al., 2019). Other frequently reported challenges include poorer driving performance, impaired cognitive abilities, compromised psychosocial functioning, lower self-confidence, and higher risk for substance abuse (Kooij et al., 2019).

*Few adults with ADHD receive appropriate treatment*

One possible explanation for poor outcomes in adults with ADHD is that relatively few individuals in this cohort receive appropriate treatment and studies have found that treatment changes are frequent (Schein et al., 2021). Barkley and colleagues (2008) reported that only one third of adults with ADHD that participated in their study had been previously diagnosed or received treatment for the disorder. Moreover, Kessler et al. (2006) reported that among adults in the National Comorbidity Survey Replication, only 10%

of participants with ADHD were receiving any type of treatment. There is an accumulating body of evidence to suggest that adults with untreated ADHD experience especially poor outcomes (Harpin et al., 2016). For example, in a meta-analysis, Shaw and colleagues (2012) compared long-term outcomes in individuals who had been treated versus not treated for ADHD. The meta-analysis comprised 351 longitudinal studies encompassing child, adolescent, and adult samples, affording a life-span view of the disorder. Specific ADHD symptoms were not included as outcomes; rather, the authors investigated individuals' functioning in a variety of key life domains. Results revealed that untreated adults with ADHD reported poorer functioning in terms of academic and occupational achievement, driving, and social functioning; increased services use (e.g., involvement with the justice system, emergency health care system, receipt of financial assistance); and higher levels of substance use/addictive behavior, antisocial behavior, and obesity as compared to adults with ADHD who received treatment (Shaw et al., 2012).

Additional analyses were conducted to determine which functional domains were most responsive to treatment. Results revealed that obesity and driving emerged as most responsive to treatment, whereas self-esteem, social functioning, and academic domains were less responsive to treatment (Shaw et al., 2012). Outcome variables identified as least responsive to treatment included substance use/addictive behavior, antisocial behavior, use of services, and occupational achievement. In addition, treatment of ADHD did not restore individuals to normative functioning in adulthood. Specifically, even those individuals with ADHD who received treatment did not evidence comparable functioning to adults without ADHD in most domains. Although individuals treated for ADHD demonstrated improvement in social and academic function relative to nontreated adults with ADHD, these individuals still remained significantly more impaired in these areas as compared to adults with no history of ADHD (Shaw et al., 2012). Unfortunately, the differential impact of specific treatment modalities (e.g., pharmacological versus behavioral) was not investigated for this study.

Relatively little outcome data are available in the adult cohort for the efficacy of different psychopharmacological treatment modalities. By way of comparison, a large body of controlled clinical trials has documented the beneficial effects of stimulant medication in improving the core symptoms of ADHD in children. Although some recent findings are suggestive of similar response in adults (Kooij et al., 2010), other studies present a more nuanced picture. A meta-analysis of 19 double-blind, placebo-controlled studies investigated the efficacy of treatment with stimulant medications relative to nonstimulant medications in the management of ADHD symptoms among adults. Findings revealed that nonstimulant medications were significantly less effective for reducing the core symptoms of ADHD as compared to long-acting stimulant medications (Faraone & Glatt, 2009). With respect to the stimulant medications included in this meta-analysis, there were no significant differences in efficacy between methylphenidate-based and amphetamine-based medications. However, findings from a recent meta-analysis revealed that amphetamine-based formulas were preferred as first-choice medications for the short-term treatment of ADHD in adults (Cortese et al., 2018).

> Psychological treatment is most effective when clients demonstrate high levels of motivation and commitment to change

The nonpharmacological treatment of adult ADHD presents significant challenges and has a growing but still relatively limited evidence base. Although young people with ADHD benefit from a variety of evidence-based nonpharmacological interventions for ADHD, including behavioral parent training, behavioral classroom management, and behavioral peer interventions (Evans et al., 2014), employing these strategies in the adult cohort is difficult as it requires consistent application of cognitive and behavioral approaches that generally include participation of a caregiver and/or authority figure. The Research Forum on Psychological Treatment for Adults with ADHD identified moderate to large effect sizes from five empirical studies (Weiss et al., 2008). However, the authors cautioned that psychological treatments, including the use of CBT, was most effective when clients demonstrated high levels of motivation and commitment to change. In a recent systematic review and meta-analysis by the Canadian ADHD Resource Alliance work group, the authors recommended CBT for reducing global, inattention, and hyperactivity/impulsivity symptoms of ADHD for adults (Tourjman et al., 2022). The work group authors indicated that their confidence in the efficacy of CBT interventions for adults with ADHD is moderate. Another meta-analysis that evaluated the long-term efficacy of psychosocial treatments, particularly CBT, for adults with ADHD revealed that treatment groups evidenced greater improvement than control groups in self-reported core symptoms of ADHD symptoms, and these gains were generally maintained for at least 12 months (López-Pinar et al., 2018).

There is some evidence to suggest that organizational-skills training among adults with ADHD may hold more promise. For example, Solanto and colleagues (2008) enrolled 30 adults with ADHD (68.4% taking medication) in an 8- or 12-week metacognitive therapy program designed to address deficits in organizational, time-management, and planning abilities. The program taught participants to use self-reinforcement to shape behavior and provided additional instruction in a variety of areas including using organizational planners, establishing priorities, setting goals, and breaking complex tasks into manageable chunks. Results revealed a large effect size (0.59) for improvement on the CAARS Inattentive subscale, on which 46.7% of the participants no longer scored in the clinical range at posttest. In addition, total scores on the BADDS, scores on subscales assessing activation, attention, effort, affect, and memory, and scores on the Organization and Planning Scale significantly improved between pre- and posttreatment. Notably, gains were made irrespective of participants' medication status. In a follow-up investigation benefiting from a randomized clinical trials design, Solanto et al. (2010) randomly assigned 88 adults with ADHD, most of whom were taking medication, to receive metacognitive therapy or supportive therapy. Results indicated that 42.2% of adults in the treatment group evidenced a favorable response to treatment, defined as at least a 30% decline in *DSM-IV* symptoms of ADHD, as compared to 12% of adults in the supportive therapy group. These findings provide support for the argument that skills-based approaches to treating ADHD among adults may hold significant benefit.

Psychosocial treatment packages that focus on conditions commonly comorbid with ADHD (e.g., depression and anxiety) have demonstrated efficacy in treating the core symptoms of ADHD as well as symptoms associated with the respective comorbid disorders (Rostain & Ramsay, 2006). Although there is evidence to suggest that a skills-training approach may be effective in ameliorating symptoms of ADHD among adults, it also is important to note that this research is in the early stages. For example, the impact of organizational-skills training on hyperactive symptoms was not investigated by Solanto and colleagues (2008, 2010). Although symptoms of inattention are more common among adults with ADHD as compared to children with ADHD, there remains a pressing need to investigate behavioral approaches to treating fidgetiness and restlessness among adults with ADHD.

Another important caveat is that no large-scale randomized clinical trials have parsed out the relative benefits of psychopharmacological treatment, psychotherapeutic intervention, and/or combined treatment among adults with ADHD. In the child ADHD cohort, results from the MTA study revealed that rates of normalization of behavior were 34% for treatment with behavior therapy, 56% for medication management, and 68% for combined treatment, suggesting an added benefit to using the combined approach (Swanson et al., 2001). Because of the chronicity of symptoms throughout the life span, as well as significant long-term impairments that can stem from inadequate treatment, clinicians should consider the use of a multimodal approach when working with adults with ADHD.

**Multimodal treatments provide many advantages relative to medication or psychosocial treatment alone**

## 4.4 Variations and Combinations of Methods

Over the years, there has been widespread interest in examining the efficacy of pharmacological and evidenced-based psychotherapeutic interventions applied separately and in combination with each other. The value of combining pharmacological and psychotherapeutic interventions to treat ADHD was established by the largest and most comprehensive clinical trial of ADHD (The MTA Cooperative Group, 1999). Including 579 participants across several sites throughout the US, the investigation clearly demonstrated the efficacy of stimulant drug therapy in reducing those symptoms associated with ADHD. However, probably the most important finding of the study is that it supported the superiority of a combined approach as compared to medication alone or treatment as usual in the community. This finding of the value of a combined approach to therapies was particularly true for those with comorbid conditions (Jensen et al., 2001) and those from more disadvantaged backgrounds when aggression was the target behavior (Rieppi et al., 2002). Further, other studies have demonstrated that a combination of behavioral interventions and stimulant medication may be as efficacious as medication used alone (Fabiano et al., 2007; Pelham et al., 2014) and is associated with improved treatment adherence (Cunill et al., 2015). As Brown and colleagues (2008) have pointed out, an advantage of the combination of a pharmacological approach employing low-dose medication combined with a behavioral intervention is that the untoward effects of medication may be tolerated more readily than higher doses of medication and that such combined therapeutic approaches may be more sustainable over the course of time.

As Evans et al. (2021) noted, one concern pertaining to the introduction of medication and psychotherapy simultaneously is that the specific contribution of each approach in the management of ADHD is uncertain. More recently, investigators have been interested in the sequencing of medication and psychotherapy to derive an optimal approach to managing ADHD. Some experts have suggested that treatment planning and sequencing of medication should be based on the individual's and family's goal in their preferences for treatment. For example, as Power and colleagues (2012) have observed, families from ethnic minority and racial backgrounds frequently have concerns about the use of medication to manage attentional and behavioral problems and obviously this is an important issue to consider in the development of treatment planning.

It is noteworthy that recent findings have suggested that the use of behavioral management employed initially, followed by the use of stimulant medication on an as needed basis, may result in enhanced outcomes relative to the initial introduction of medication as the sole treatment modality. Pelham et al. (2014) have argued that family engagement, which is frequently required in behavior management, was greater when behavior management was implemented initially relative to stimulant medication. Obviously, the ultimate goal of any intervention is the individual's functional outcome across settings (in the employment setting and at home) and thus intervention planning should always include the fostering of strong relationships with significant others and family members. It also should be noted that while medication alone would be difficult to justify given the evidence of the MTA investigation (The MTA Cooperative Group, 1999), as Evans et al. (2021) have highlighted, medication may facilitate coping and also promote success across settings including the work setting.

In another investigation that examined the impact of multimodal therapies among adults with ADHD, Safren and associates (2005) introduced a cognitive-behavioral intervention to adults with ADHD who were designated as stable on medication, yet who also continued to experience significant impairments associated with the disorder. Participants were assigned randomly to receive either CBT in addition to pharmacotherapy or to continue to receive pharmacotherapy alone. Cognitive therapy included psychoeducation about ADHD and effective organizational strategies, learning skills to maximize distractibility, and cognitive restructuring to manage adaptive thought processes during stressful experiences. Findings from the study revealed that participants in the pharmacotherapy combined with the cognitive-behavioral intervention demonstrated reductions in symptoms related to ADHD relative to participants in the pharmacotherapy alone group. Finally, those participants who received CBT were found to report fewer symptoms of depression and anxiety relative to those who received only medication.

In a similar investigation to that of Safren and associates (2005), Bramham and associates (2009) conducted a study adding CBT to pharmacotherapy in 61 adults with ADHD. In one group, participants completed day-long group cognitive therapy sessions and this group was compared to a wait-list control group receiving only medication. The cognitive therapy group received psychoeducational training, frustration tolerance and anger management, understanding thought–behavior relationships to manage issues related to mood and self-esteem, social skills training, and, finally, time-management and problem-solving skills. Not surprisingly, findings revealed that the cognitive therapy intervention resulted in participants' self-rated improvements on measures of their knowledge and understanding of ADHD. Moreover, improvement also were evidenced on participants' self-ratings of self-esteem and self-efficacy. No treatment effects were revealed for measures of depressive symptoms and anxiety. Unfortunately, the study did not assess specific symptoms of ADHD and, thus, the effects of the intervention on ADHD specifically cannot be addressed.

The corpus of evidence clearly suggests that the combination of pharmacological and psychotherapeutic interventions is likely effective in the management of adult ADHD. In fact, the European Consensus Statement on Diagnosis and Treatment of Adult ADHD has recommended multimodal treatments for ADHD (Kooij et al., 2010). Various therapeutic interventions included in the algorithm for this approach include psychoeducation of ADHD and comorbid disorders, pharmacotherapy for ADHD and comorbid disorders, coaching, CBT in both individual and group formats, and, finally, family therapy (Kooji et al., 2010).

Unfortunately, no large-scale randomized clinical trials have examined the efficacy of multimodal treatments with ADHD. Extant literature also has failed to address a number of concerns related to the use of multimodal therapies to manage individuals with ADHD in the community. It is noteworthy that in both Rostain and Ramsay (2006) and the Safren and colleagues (2005) studies of multimodal treatments among adults with ADHD, potential participants were eliminated with comorbid conditions of moderate to severe depression and current substance abuse. Given the high comorbidity associated with adult ADHD, much more research is needed that examines multimodal interventions for adults with ADHD and other comorbid conditions to have more enhanced external validity.

The search for empirically validated cost-effective and efficient treatment protocols is necessary as we seek the best management approaches for ADHD in adults. In addition, the appropriate sequencing of treatment will be necessary as we embark on multimodal treatments for adults. Further, research related to consumer satisfaction with pharmacological and psychotherapeutic interventions will be necessary. Given the ongoing time commitments associated with psychosocial therapies and the seeming lack of available resources given the shortage of mental health providers after the COVID-19 pandemic, it stands to reason that psychosocial interventions may be less desirable than pharmacological therapies for adults. Moreover, given adults' more developed cognitive schema relative to their pediatric counterparts, it may be reasoned that adults are better able to make use of psychosocial therapies such as CBT (Safren et al., 2005). In support of this notion, Rostain and Ramsay (2006) have argued that CBT to manage ADHD among adults provided a top-down method of managing the disorder by teaching these individuals executive skills and coping strategies thereby not being solely reliant on a bottom-up approach associated with medication as the only treatment modality for the disorder. It is thus reasoned that a multimodal treatment plan may provide a more durable treatment plan for these individuals thereby reducing their need for ongoing pharmacotherapy. Clearly, additional research must be mounted to evaluate the efficacy of such approaches, consumer satisfaction associated with such approaches, and to test whether specific interventions are more efficacious and viable for specific types of ADHD and comorbid groups.

## 4.5 Problems in Carrying Out the Treatments

Treatment of ADHD in adults presents unique challenges to the clinician (Geffen & Forster, 2018) and often requires an individualized approach. Formal treatment guidelines for adult ADHD have not been developed in the US. In addition, comorbid mental health disorders are highly prevalent in adults with ADHD and can significantly complicate treatment (Mattingly et al., 2021). There is evidence to suggest differential effects of psychostimulants on individuals with and without comorbid psychiatric conditions (Stevens et al., 2013). For example, medications commonly prescribed for ADHD may be less effective and/or exacerbate symptoms in individuals with comorbid conditions such as depression, anxiety, or substance abuse/dependence (Torgersen et al., 2008). There is some but not robust data in the adult ADHD literature to guide the clinician when seeking to determine in which comorbidities, and under what circumstances, psychostimulant medications are contraindicated (Geffen & Forster, 2018). Therefore, clinicians are advised to carefully monitor patients treated with stimulant medication for exacerbation of comorbid symptoms and to work closely with prescribing professionals to communicate concerns about preexisting or potentially worsening comorbid conditions. Moreover, the therapist must use their clinical judgment to determine whether psychotherapeutic or pharmacological interventions for comorbid disorders should precede ADHD treatment (Geffen & Forster, 2018). If ADHD is felt to be the patient's primary diagnosis but comorbidities are also a concern, clinicians may choose to adopt the CBT treatment protocols developed by Rostain and Ramsay (2006) and Safren et al. (2005). Notably, each of these protocols includes components to treat secondary comorbidities common in individuals with ADHD (e.g., depression, anxiety). However, treatment of substance abuse or dependence should generally precede any ADHD interventions (Kooij et al., 2010).

Another significant challenge encountered by clinicians working with adults with ADHD is low levels of medication adherence. Findings from a study that investigated stimulant treatment adherence in adult ADHD patients found that less than 12% were adherent to medication (O'Callaghan, 2014). Some experts have suggested that low rates of stimulant medication response in adult ADHD patients may reflect suboptimal treatment adherence in this cohort as a whole (Safren et al., 2005).

Effective management of ADHD can be time and labor intensive; therefore, it is not surprising that some adults with ADHD struggle with treatment adherence. In addition, adults with ADHD, as compared to children with ADHD, are less likely to have individuals in their lives (e.g., parents) who can provide significant assistance in the management of their condition. Even if these individuals are available, some adults with ADHD may not be comfortable disclosing their condition and/or receiving help. Additional correlates of nonadherence may include executive dysfunction or stigma regarding an ADHD diagnosis or treatment with medication. If beliefs about psychotropic medications and/or stigma regarding ADHD are negatively impacting adherence to treatment, clinicians should provide patients with adequate psychoeducation regarding their condition and be open to discussing any potential concerns with respect to treatment options. Clinicians also should proactively seek to problem solve issues (e.g., financial concerns, organizational difficulties) that may impact patients' ability to adhere to medication and/or psychosocial interventions. When feasible, other responsible individuals (e.g., spouses/partners, siblings, or other treating professionals) should be encouraged to participate in a collective effort to assist adults with ADHD with adherence to treatment. Lastly, the clinician should closely consider a patient's strengths, deficits, and resources when engaging in treatment planning.

> Lack of adherence to treatment by the adult is common and can compromise successful treatment

## 4.6 Multicultural Issues

Cultural and diversity considerations are a critical and core component in any clinical evaluation and treatment planning efforts, including those for ADHD. Unfortunately, individuals of color and those from socially disadvantaged backgrounds are not always included in adult ADHD diagnosis and treatment research. In fact, very little is known about cultural or ethnic diversity in adult ADHD (Waite & Ramsay, 2010). Equally problematic is that the current *DSM-5* ADHD symptoms were based on observations of youth who were primarily White male US schoolchildren (Conners, 2000).

It is only more recently that research has started to examine in depth the impact of cultural and diversity factors on ADHD diagnosis and treatment effectiveness for adults. Clinicians should therefore be mindful and examine if research or clinical guidelines support utilization or modifications for individuals from certain cultural groups. Some recommendations have been published for working with different cultural groups. For example, Rostain, Ramsay, and Waite (2015) note that, for some Black or African American adults with ADHD, modifying CBT for ADHD to be culturally congruent might include incorporation of the individual's intergenerational system. The authors also highlight that Black or African American adults with ADHD have lower stimulant use for a variety of reasons, potentially impacting first-line treatment recommendations for these individuals. Rostain, Ramsay, and Waite (2015) suggest that when clinicians treat Latino adults with ADHD, they should spend additional time on ADHD education and rapport building due to reduced knowledge about ADHD and increased mistrust of health care providers relative to those from other cultures.

The extant research on potential gender differences for pharmacological treatments for ADHD are inconsistent (Williamson & Johnston, 2015), potentially due to approximately one third of studies not reporting data by gender (Surman et al., 2013). Similarly, less than one fourth of psychosocial treatments examined differential impacts by gender (Williamson & Johnston, 2015). Clinicians should also be mindful that ADHD was initially defined primarily around male samples.

There is still much to be done with respect to multicultural considerations for adult ADHD treatment. Diagnostic and treatment recommendations often only consider one aspect of an individual's cultural identity. In line with recent American Psychological Association guidelines (2017), treatment providers should conceptualize their cases and treatment utilizing an intersectional framework. For example, individuals from one cultural group may be quite different from one another due to SES (e.g., Rostain, Diaz, & Pedraza, 2015). Clinicians should therefore consider all aspects of an individual's identity, the intersectionality of these identities, and the extant literature on treatments for adults with ADHD to design an optimal treatment approach. As research that includes multicultural factors continues to be published, clinicians can look to the literature for additional guidance on treating diverse adults with ADHD.

# 5

# Case Vignettes

## Julie (college student)

Julie is a 19-year-old Caucasian student in the second term of her first year at college. Although she reported expending a great deal of effort in her coursework, Julie had received failing grades on her midterms in two history courses. She made an appointment at the counseling center on campus to discuss her academic difficulties. Julie had always been interested in history and had been considering a career in academia but, after her struggles with her history classes, she wondered whether she needed to change her major and professional plans. Julie described an active social life and has felt the strain of competing academic and social pressures.

During elementary school, junior high, and high school, Julie consistently struggled in class with inattention, distractibility, and disorganization of materials. She would often daydream during class and her teachers needed to frequently redirect her attention back to the course material. Fortunately, Julie attended a small private school with a low student–teacher ratio, so her teachers were able to provide her with a significant amount of support for staying focused and engaged during class. Julie was always seated next to a peer that could help her stay on task and repeat instructions that she missed.

Julie reports having ongoing difficulties with organization. She noted trouble keeping track of important papers, and often losing clothing or other items. Julie's mother was very involved in her life during the elementary and secondary school years. Julie reports that her mom helped her maintain a daily assignment book, organize her class materials, clean her room, and complete homework. Without her mom's daily support, Julie found the first term of college to be much more challenging than high school, and her academic performance in college has been a disappointment to her. However, during her initial term, she attended the college's freshman seminar program, and received quite a bit of individual attention, which she says was quite helpful. During the current term, she is enrolled in two large lecture classes and two smaller seminar classes. Although some of the material from lectures is accessible in the textbooks, Julie feels she has a difficulty time maintaining her attention during the lectures and it is difficult taking adequate notes. She feels competent during small interactive classes and has received high grades for her assignments in these classes but has failed the multiple-choice tests that comprise a major portion of her grade in both courses. Julie is especially upset about this because she believes that, in some cases, she understood the material that appeared on the tests, but could not recall it at the time.

Julie also describes some strain in balancing her social life with her academic objectives, and notes that her academic failures have influenced her sense of identity. In high school, she had a group of friends who tended to socialize together. In college, Julie has made several new friends in her dormitory and in her classes but finds that she often forgets social events that she had planned. Although at times she has forgotten or cancelled social plans because of her schoolwork, she describes being so upset about her academic difficulties that she has increased her socializing and feels that spending time with friends offers a positive escape from her academic concerns. Julie has indicated that she is very demoralized by her poor academic performance. She explained that she feels "like a failure" and that her sense of herself as a capable student has been seriously disrupted.

One of Julie's friends has ADHD and takes stimulant medication. This friend offered her a dose of the medication, which she tried before a history lecture. She noticed that her concentration and grasp of that lecture's material seemed to come more easily than usual. Julie wondered whether ADHD might be responsible for some of her difficulties. Her goal in coming to the counseling center was to obtain a referral for an evaluation for ADHD and to determine whether medication might be helpful for her academic difficulties.

At the office of a private practitioner, Julie participated in a full assessment for ADHD, which included the CAA-DID *DSM-IV*, the Behavior Rating Inventory of Executive Function–Adult self-report form (BRIEF-A), the WAIS-IV, the Wechsler Individual Achievement Test – third edition (WIAT-III), the Wechsler Memory Scales – third edition (WMS-III), and the CPT. Julie's mother was able to provide information in an interview over the phone about her childhood behaviors. She also completed a checklist of Julie's symptoms and faxed some of Julie's old school report cards to the counseling center. Julie's mother and several of her high school teachers identified her difficulties with organization and a tendency to be easily distracted. Julie also noted these difficulties herself during the clinical interview with the CAA-DID. In addition, findings from the BRIEF-A also revealed significant problems with working memory and organization of materials. Her WMS-III, WAIS-IV, and CPT scores were consistent with those of individuals with ADHD. Following this assessment, Julie was referred to the staff psychiatrist at the college counseling center, who prescribed Adderall to target her attentional difficulties. She also had three counseling sessions at the student health center, which used CBT to address her negative thoughts around her coursework and its effects on her identity. The counseling sessions also used behavioral strategies to help Julie take the initiative to form study groups for her history classes, which helped contribute to her improved performance in those courses.

Julie's case is typical of many new college students who managed to succeed during the elementary and secondary school years with a high level of parent and teacher support, but who struggle to adjust to more demanding academic and social expectations during college without these daily supports. This type of student is unlikely to have received a diagnosis of ADHD before reaching college but may be helped by psychosocial and pharmacological interventions.

## Peter (adult)

Peter is a 34-year-old Black male who works in software development. He describes himself as having significant attention issues and feels that his grades in school were seriously compromised by his difficulties with concentration and staying on task. He also described being "fidgety" and having had trouble sitting still for long periods of time. Until Peter was diagnosed with ADHD in the ninth grade, his parents repeatedly chastised him for what they perceived as his lack of motivation and effort. Peter began taking stimulant medication in the ninth grade and found that it helped his ADHD symptoms of inattention, but that he still had trouble controlling his impulsivity. He continued taking the medication in college, but stopped after college when his work environments did not necessitate the same sorts of prolonged attention that had been necessary for his academic coursework.

Peter has worked at the same company for 6 years. When he began to work for his current employer, it had been a start-up company. Peter's job involved multiple tasks, including establishing the structure and framework for software systems, testing his company's products, developing new versions of the software, backing up the software periodically, writing scripts to automate deployment, and creating the user interface. With only four coworkers, Peter's role was rather fluid, and he "wore multiple hats." He enjoyed the variety in his work and the continued interaction with his colleagues. Peter was able to switch tasks according to his ideas and interests. The company became quite successful, and Peter felt capable and proud of his work and accomplishments.

As the company grew, Peter's job description became more specific. He was made the manager of a particular subarea. His new job demanded that he focus exclusively on release control – making sure that there are no bugs in the current version of the company's software. Peter has begun to get quite bored at work and finds that his concentration is wandering. He finds himself taking many breaks throughout the day. In addition, Peter cannot help working on projects to which he is not assigned. Though many of his coworkers appreciate his unsolicited feedback, others do not, and the work in his own department has not been up to his usual performance. Though on one level, Peter is aware that his ADHD may be related to his current difficulties, he has noticed that he has begun to view himself as lazy and unsuccessful, and to reexperience some of the negative messages about his character that he experienced while growing up. He has begun to feel rather demoralized and depressed, and notes that he is not as interested in spending time with his girlfriend, his friends, and his family as he used to be.

Peter made an appointment for psychotherapy to address his depressive feelings and to discuss whether he should resume taking medication for ADHD. His assessment included neuropsychological measures, including the WAIS-III and the CPT. It also included an extensive interview regarding Peter's employment history that included his relationships with colleagues and bosses, his work satisfaction among different tasks and jobs, and his interests and goals. The results of the assessment indicated that Peter had many of the typical neuropsychological correlates of ADHD. From his responses, it became clear that Peter excels in situations where his responsibilities span several domains and require that he integrate these topic areas. He also enjoys work that promises continued challenges and a degree of novelty.

Peter's therapy used a coaching approach that focused on teaching him coping and problem-solving skills for identified problems. Eventually, he was able to rework his position within the company to be more like his initial one, and again experienced interest and satisfaction at work and an alleviation of his depressive symptoms.

# 6

# Further Reading

Barkley, R. A. (2010). *Taking charge of adult ADHD*. Guilford Press.
Provides adults with step-by-step strategies for managing symptoms and reducing their harmful impact. Readers get hands-on self-assessment tools and skills-building exercises, plus clear answers to frequently asked questions about medications and other treatments. Specific techniques are presented for overcoming challenges in critical areas where people with the disorder often struggle – work, finances, relationships, and more.

Barkley, R. A. (2014). *Attention-deficit hyperactivity disorder: A handbook for diagnosis and treatment* (4th ed.). Guilford Press.
Widely regarded as the standard clinical reference for ADHD. It provides knowledge about ADHD in children, adolescents, and adults, including conceptualizations and evidence-based guidelines for assessment, diagnosis, and treatment approaches in a range of settings. The book examines the impact of the disorder across functional domains such as behavior, learning, school and vocational outcomes, and health. Given the breadth of relevant topics covered, this resource is instrumental for both researchers and clinicians.

Boissiere, P. (2018). *Thriving with adult ADHD: Skills to strengthen executive functioning*. Althea Press.
Offers daily strategies to help readers succeed with adult ADHD. The book focuses on executive-functioning skills including focus, organization, and stress management. Chapters contain information, assessments, and evidence-based exercises to help build mental skills to address the challenges associated with ADHD.

Brown, T. E. (2017). *Outside the box: Rethinking ADD/ADHD in children and adults – A practical guide*. American Psychiatric Association.
For professionals working with individuals with ADHD as well as for those experiencing the challenges of having ADHD. The book describes ADHD across the life span and provides useful clinical vignettes while also debunking common misunderstandings about ADHD.

Hallowell, E. M., & Ratey, J. J. (2021). *ADHD 2.0: New science and essential strategies for thriving with distraction – From childhood through adulthood*. Ballantine Books.
Provides updates on recent research developments, including a clearer understanding of the ADHD brain. The authors describe the positives and negatives associated with ADHD and offer new strategies and lifestyle hacks for thriving with ADHD.

# 7

# References

Adler, L., Kessler, R. C., Spencer, T., & World Health Organization. (2013). *Adult ADHD Self-Report Scale (ASRS-v1. 1) symptom checklist instructions*. World Health Organization.

Adler, L. A., Spencer, T. J., & Wilens, T. E. (Eds.). (2015). *Attention-deficit hyperactivity disorder in adults and children*. Cambridge University Press.

Advokat, C., & Scheithauer, M. (2013). Attention-deficit hyperactivity disorder (ADHD) stimulant medications as cognitive enhancers. *Frontiers in Neuroscience*, 7. https://doi.org/10.3389/fnins.2013.00082

Ambrosini, P. J. (2000). Historical development and present status of the schedule for affective disorders and schizophrenia for school-age children (K-SADS). *Journal of the American Academy of Child & Adolescent Psychiatry, 39*(1), 49–58. https://doi.org/10.1097/00004583-200001000-0001

American Psychiatric Association (APA). (2000). *Diagnostic and statistical manual of mental disorders* (4th ed., text rev.). https://doi.org/10.1176/appi.books.9780890423349

American Psychiatric Association (APA). (2013). *Diagnostic and statistical manual of mental disorders* (5th ed.). https://doi/10.1176/appi.books.9780890425596

American Psychiatric Association (APA). (2022). *Diagnostic and statistical manual of mental disorders* (5th ed., text rev.). https://doi.org/10.1176/appi.books.9780890425787

American Psychological Association. (2017). *Multicultural guidelines: An ecological approach to context, identity, and intersectionality,* 2017. http://www.apa.org/about/policy/multicultural-guidelines.aspx

Arnold, L. E., Hodgkins, P., Kahle, J., Madhoo, M., & Kewley, G. (2020). Long-term outcomes of ADHD: Academic achievement and performance. *Journal of Attention Disorders, 24*(1), 73–85. https://doi.org/10.1177/1087054714566076

Asarnow, R. F., Newman, N., Weiss, R. E., & Su, E. (2021). Association of attention-deficit/hyperactivity disorder diagnoses with pediatric traumatic brain injury: A meta-analysis. *JAMA Pediatrics, 175*(10), 1009–1016. https://doi.org/10.1001/jamapediatrics.2021.2033

Asherson, P., Akehurst, R., Kooij, J. J., Huss, M., Beusterien, K., Sasané, R., Gholizadeh, S., & Hodgkins, P. (2012). Under diagnosis of adult ADHD cultural influences and societal burden. *Journal of Attention Disorders, 16*(Suppl. 5), 20S–38S. https://doi.org/10.1177/1087054711435360

Asherson, P., Buitelaar, J., Faraone, S. V., & Rohde, L. A. (2016). Adult attention-deficit hyperactivity disorder: Key conceptual issues. *Lancet Psychiatry, 3*(6), 568–578. https://doi.org/10.1016/s2215-0366(16)30032-3

Barkley, R. A. (1997). Behavioral inhibition, sustained attention, and executive functions: Constructing a unifying theory of ADHD. *Psychological Bulletin, 121*(1), 65–94. https://doi.org/10.1037/0033-2909.121.1.65

Barkley, R. A. (2011). *Barkley Adult ADHD Rating Scale-IV (BAARS-IV)*. Guilford Press.

Barkley, R. A. (2015). *Attention-deficit hyperactivity disorder: A handbook for diagnosis and treatment* (4th ed.). Guilford Press.

# 7. References

Barkley, R. A. (2019). Neuropsychological testing is not useful in the diagnosis of ADHD: Stop it (or prove it)! *ADHD Report, 27*(2), 1-8. https://doi.org/10.1521/adhd.2019.27.2.1

Barkley R. A. (2020). ADHD adversely impacts health, mortality risk, and estimated life expectancy by adulthood. *The ADHD Report, 28*(4), 1-4.

Barkley, R. A. (2022). *Treating ADHD in children and adolescents: What every clinician needs to know*. Guilford Press.

Barkley, R. A., & Benton, C. M. (2021). *Taking charge of adult ADHD: Proven strategies to succeed at work, at home, and in relationships* (2nd ed.). Guilford Press.

Barkley, R. A., & Fischer, M. (2010). The unique contribution of emotional impulsiveness to impairment in major life activities in hyperactive children as adults. *Journal of the American Academy of Child and Adolescent Psychiatry, 49*(5), 503-513. https://doi.org/10.1097/00004583-201005000-0001

Barkley, R. A., Murphy, K. R., & Fischer, M. (2010). *ADHD in adults: What the science says*. Guilford Press.

Barkley, R. A., & Peters, H. (2012). The earliest reference to ADHD in the medical literature? Melchior Adam Weikard's description in 1775 of "attention deficit" (mangel der aufmerksamkeit, attentio volubilis). *Journal of Attention Disorders, 16*, 623-630. https://doi.org/10.1177/1087054711432309

Bax, A. C., Bard, D. E., Cuffe, S. P., McKeown, R. E., & Wolraich, M. L. (2019). The association between race/ethnicity and socioeconomic factors and the diagnosis and treatment of children with attention-deficit hyperactivity disorder. *Journal of Developmental & Behavioral Pediatrics, 40*(2), 81-91. https://doi.org/10.1097/dbp.0000000000000626

Beck, A. T., & Steer, R. A. (1993). *Manual for the Beck Anxiety Inventory*. Psychological Corporation.

Beck, A. T., Steer, R. A., & Brown, G. K. (1996). *Manual for Beck Depression Inventory-II (BDI-II)*. Psychological Corporation.

Benson, K., Flory, K., Humphreys, K. L., & Lee, S. S. (2015). Misuse of stimulant medication among college students: A comprehensive review and meta-analysis. *Clinical Child and Family Psychology Review, 18*(1), 50-76. https://doi.org/10.1007/s10567-014-0177-z

Berg, E. A. (1948). A simple objective technique for measuring flexibility in thinking. *Journal of General Psychology, 39*, 15-22. https://doi.org/10.1080/00221309.1948.9918159

Bernardi, S., Faraone, S. V., Cortese, S., Kerridge, B. T., Pallanti, S., Wang, S., & Blanco, C. (2012). The lifetime impact of attention deficit hyperactivity disorder: Results from the National Epidemiologic Survey on Alcohol and Related Conditions (NESARC). *Psychological Medicine, 42*(4), 875-887. https://doi.org/10.1017/S003329171100153X

Biederman, J., Monuteaux, M. C., Mick, E., Spencer, T., Wilens, T. E., Silva, J. M., Snyder, L. E., & Faraone, S. V. (2006). Young adult outcome of attention deficit hyperactivity disorder: A controlled 10-year follow-up study. *Psychological Medicine, 36*(2), 167-179. https://doi.org/10.1017/S0033291705006410

Biederman, J., Petty, C. R., O'Connor, K. B., Hyder, L. L., & Faraone, S. V. (2012). Predictors of persistence in girls with attention deficit hyperactivity disorder: Results from an 11-year controlled follow-up study. *Acta Psychiatrica Scandinavica, 125*(2), 147-156. https://doi.org/10.1111/j.1600-0447.2011.01797.x

Blackman, G. L., Ostrander, R., & Herman, K. C. (2005). Children with ADHD and depression: A multisource, multimethod assessment of clinical, social, and academic functioning. *Journal of Attention Disorders, 8*(4), 195-207. https://doi.org/10.1177/1087054705278777

Bramham, J., Young, S., Bickerdike, A., Spain, D., McCartan, D., & Xenitidis, K. (2009). Evaluation of group cognitive behavioral therapy for adults with ADHD. *Journal of Attention Disorders, 12*(5), 434-441. https://doi.org/10.1177/1087054708314596

Breda, V., Cerqueira, R. O., Ceolin, G., Koning, E., Fabe, J., McDonald, A., Gomes, F. A., & Brietzke, E. (2022). Is there a place for dietetic interventions in adult ADHD? *Progress in Neuro-Psychopharmacology and Biological Psychiatry, 19*, 110613. https://doi.org/10.1016/j.pnpbp.2022.110613

Brown, R. T. (in press). Pharmacotherapy. In B. B. Brown & M. J. Prinstein (Eds.), *Encyclopedia of adolescence*. Elsevier.

Brown, R. T. (2018). Pediatric pharmacology and psychopharmacology. In M. C. Roberts & R. G. Steele (Eds.), *Handbook of pediatric psychology* (pp. 161–178, 5th ed.). Guilford.

Brown, R. T., Antonuccio, D. O., DuPaul, G. J., Fristad, M., King, C. A., Leslie, L. K., & Vitiello, B. (2008). *Childhood mental health disorders: Evidence base and contextual factors for psychosocial, psychopharmacological and combined interventions*. American Psychological Association.

Brown, T. E. (1996). *Brown Attention-Deficit Disorder Scales*. Psychological Corporation.

Brown, T. E. (2018). *Brown Executive Function/Attention Scales (Brown EF/A Scales)*. Pearson.

Brown, T. E., & Gammon, G. D. (1991). *The Brown Attention Activation Disorder Scale: Protocol for clinical use*. Yale University.

Bukstein, O. G. (2012). Attention deficit hyperactivity disorder and substance use disorders. *Current Topics in Behavioral Neurosciences, 9*, 145–172. https://doi.org/10.1007/7854_2011_148

Bussing, R., Zima, B. T., Gary, F. A., & Garvan, C. W. (2003). Barriers to detection, help-seeking, and service use for children with ADHD symptoms. *The Journal of Behavioral Health Services & Research, 30*(2), 176–189. https://doi.org/10.1007/BF02289806

Chan, Y. F., Dennis, M. L., & Funk, R. R. (2008). Prevalence and comorbidity of major internalizing and externalizing problems among adolescents and adults presenting to substance abuse treatment. *Journal of substance abuse treatment, 34*(1), 14–24. https://doi.org/10.1016/j.jsat.2006.12.031

Chen, Q., Brikell, I., Lichtenstein, P., Serlachius, E., Kuja-Halkola, R., Sandin, S., & Larsson, H. (2017). Familial aggregation of attention-deficit/hyperactivity disorder. *Journal of Child Psychology and Psychiatry, 58*(3), 231–239. https://doi.org/10.1111/jcpp.12616

Chronis-Tuscano, A., Molina, B. S., Pelham, W. E., Applegate, B., Dahlke, A., Overmyer, M., & Lahey, B. B. (2010). Very early predictors of adolescent depression and suicide attempts in children with attention-deficit/hyperactivity disorder. *Archives of General Psychiatry, 67*(10), 1044–1051. https://doi.org/10.1001/archgenpsychiatry.2010.127

Chung, T., & Bachrach, R. L. (2021). Substance use problems. In R. J. Prinstein, E. A. Youngstrom, E. J. Mash, & R. A. Barkley (Eds.), *Treatment of disorders in childhood and adolescence* (pp. 661–703). Guilford Press.

Chung, W., Jiang, S. F., Paksarian, D., Nikolaidis, A., Castellanos, F. X., Merikangas, K. R., & Milham, M. P. (2019). Trends in the prevalence and incidence of attention-deficit/hyperactivity disorder among adults and children of different racial and ethnic groups. *JAMA Network Open, 2*(11), e1914344–e1914344. https://doi.org/10.1001/jamanetworkopen.2019.14344

Conners, C. K. (2000). Attention-deficit/hyperactivity disorder: Historical development and overview. *Journal of Attention Disorders, 3*(4), 173–191. https://doi.org/10.1177/108705470000300401

Conners, C. K., Erhardt, D., & Sparrow, E. P. (1999). *Conners' Adult ADHD Rating Scales: Technical manual*. Multi-Health Systems.

Conners, C. K., & Staff, M. (2014). *Conners' Continuous Performance Test (Conners' CPT 3)*. MHS Assessments.

Connor, D. F., & Doerfler, L. A. (2008). ADHD with comorbid oppositional defiant disorder or conduct disorder: Discrete or nondistinct disruptive behavior disorders?

*Journal of Attention Disorders, 12*(2), 126–134. https://doi.org/10.1177/1087054707308486

Cortese, S. (2012). The neurobiology and genetics of attention-deficit/hyperactivity disorder (ADHD): What every clinician should know. *European Journal of Paediatric Neurology, 16*(5), 422–433. https://doi.org/10.1016/j.ejpn.2012.01.009

Cortese, S., Adamo, N., Del Giovane, C., Mohr-Jensen, C., Hayes, A. J., Carucci, S., Atkinson, L. Z., Tessari, L., Banaschewski, T., Coghill, D., Hollis, C., Simonoff, E., Zuddas, A., Barbui, C., Purgato, M., Steinhausen, H. C., Shokraneh, F., Xia, J., & Cipriani, A. (2018). Comparative efficacy and tolerability of medications for attention-deficit hyperactivity disorder in children, adolescents, and adults: A systematic review and network meta-analysis. *Lancet Psychiatry, 5*(9), 727–738. https://doi.org/10.1016/s2215-0366(18)30269-4

Cunill, R., Castells, X., Tobias, A., & Capellà, D. (2015). Efficacy, safety and variability in pharmacotherapy for adults with attention deficit hyperactivity disorder: A meta-analysis and meta-regression in over 9000 patients. *Psychopharmacology, 233*(2), 187–197. https://doi.org/10.1007/s00213-015-4099-3

Delis, D. C., Kaplan, E., & Kramer, J. (2001). *Delis-Kaplan Executive Function System*. Psychological Corporation.

Delis, D. C., Kramer, J. H., Kaplan, E., & Ober, B. A. (2017). *California Verbal Learning Test-3* (3rd ed.). Psychological Corporation.

Del-Ponte, B., Quinte, G. C., Cruz, S., Grellert, M., & Santos, I. S. (2019). Dietary patterns and attention deficit hyperactivity disorder (ADHD): A systematic review and meta-analysis. *Journal of Affective Disorders, 252*(1), 160–173. https://doi.org/https://doi.org/10.1016/j.jad.2019.04.061

Derogatis, L. R. (1975). *The Symptom Checklist 90 – Revised*. NCS Assessments.

Doshi, J. A., Hodgkins, P., Kahle, J., Sikirica, V., Cangelosi, M. J., Setyawan, J., Erder, M. H., & Neumann, P. J. (2012). Economic impact of childhood and adult attention-deficit/hyperactivity disorder in the United States. *Journal of the American Academy of Child & Adolescent Psychiatry, 51*(10), 990–1002.e2. https://doi.org/10.1016/j.jaac.2012.07.008

Drechsler, R., Brem, S., Brandeis, D., Grünblatt, E., Berger, G., & Walitza, S. (2020). ADHD: Current concepts and treatments in children and adolescents. *Neuropediatrics, 51*(5), 315–335. https://doi.org/10.1055/s-0040-1701658

DuPaul, G. J., Gormley, M. J., & Laracy, S. D. (2013). Comorbidity of LD and ADHD: Implications of DSM-5 for assessment and treatment. *Journal of Learning Disabilities, 46*(1), 43–51. https://doi.org/10.1177/0022219412464351

DuPaul, G. J., Power, T. J., Anastopoulos, A. D., & Reid, R. (2016). *ADHD Rating Scale-5 for Children and Adolescents: Checklists, norms, and clinical interpretation*. Guilford Press.

Elliott, J., Johnston, A., Husereau, D., Kelly, S. E., Eagles, C., Charach, A., Hsieh, S. C., Bai, Z., Hossain, A., Skidmore, B., Tsakonas, E., Chojecki, D., Mamdani, M., & Wells, G. A. (2020). Pharmacologic treatment of attention deficit hyperactivity disorder in adults: A systematic review and network meta-analysis. *PLoS One, 15*(10), e0240584. https://doi.org/10.1371/journal.pone.0240584

Epstein, J. N., Johnson, D. E., & Conners, C. K. (2001). *The Conners' Adult ADHD Diagnostic Interview for DSM-IV (CAADID)*. Multi-Health Systems.

Epstein, J. N., & Kollins, S. H. (2006). Psychometric properties of an adult ADHD diagnostic interview. *Journal of Attention Disorders, 9*(3), 504–514. https://doi.org/10.1177/1087054705283575

Evans, S. W., Owens, J. S., & Bunford, N. (2014). Evidence-based psychosocial treatments for children and adolescents with attention-deficit/hyperactivity disorder. *Journal of Clinical Child and Adolescent Psychology, 43*(4), 527–551. https://doi.org/10.1080/15374416.2013.850700

Evans, S. W., Owens, J. S., & Power, T. J. (2021). Attention-deficit/hyperactivity disorder. In R. J. Prinstein, E. A. Youngstrom, E. J. Mash, & R. A. Barkley (Eds.), *Treatment of disorders in childhood and adolescence* (pp. 47–101). Guilford Press.

Evans, S. W., Owens, J. S., Wymbs, B. T., & Ray, A. R. (2018). Evidence-based psychosocial treatments for children and adolescents with attention deficit/hyperactivity disorder. *Journal of Clinical Child and Adolescent Psychology, 47*(2), 157–198. https://doi.org/10.1080/15374416.2017.1390757

Fabiano, G. A., Pelham, W. E., Jr., Gnagy, E. M., Burrows-MacLean, L., Coles, E. K., Chacko, A., Wymbs, B. T., Walker, K. S., Arnold, F., Garefino, A., Keenan, J. K., Onyango, A. N., Hoffman, M. T., Massetti, G. M., & Robb, J. A. (2007). The single and combined effects of multiple intensities of behavior modification and methylphenidate for children with attention deficit hyperactivity disorder in a classroom setting. *School Psychology Review, 36*(2), 195–216. https://doi.org/10.1080/02796015.2007.12087940

Faraone, S. V., & Glatt, S. J. (2009). A comparison of the efficacy of medications for adult attention-deficit/hyperactivity disorder using meta-analysis of effect sizes. *Journal of Clinical Psychiatry, 71*(6), 754–763. https://doi.org/10.4088/jcp.08m04902pur

Faraone, S. V., & Larsson, H. (2019). Genetics of attention deficit hyperactivity disorder. *Molecular Psychiatry, 24*(4), 562–575. https://doi.org/10.1038/s41380-018-0070-0

Farhat, L. C., Flores, J. M., Behling, E., Avila-Quintero, V. J., Lombroso, A., Cortese, S., Polanczyk, G. V., & Bloch, M. H. (2022). The effects of stimulant dose and dosing strategy on treatment outcomes in attention-deficit/hyperactivity disorder in children and adolescents: A meta-analysis. *Molecular Psychiatry, 27*(3), 1562–1572. https://doi.org/10.1038/s41380-021-01391-9

Fayyad, J., Sampson, N. A., Hwang, I., Adamowski, T., Aguilar-Gaxiola, S., Al-Hamzawi, A., Andrade, L. H., Borges, G., de Girolamo, G., Florescu, S., Gureje, O., Haro, J. M., Hu, C., Karam, E. G., Lee, S., Navarro-Mateu, F., O'Neill, S., Pennell, B. E., Piazza, M., ... Kessler, R. C. (2017). The descriptive epidemiology of DSM-IV adult ADHD in the World Health Organization world mental health surveys. *ADHD Attention Deficit and Hyperactivity Disorders, 9*(1), 47–65. https://doi.org/10.1007/s12402-016-0208-3

Fernandez, M. A., & Eyberg, S. M. (2009). Predicting treatment and follow-up attrition in parent–child interaction therapy. *Journal of Abnormal Child Psychology, 37*, 431–441. https://doi.org/10.1007/s10802-008-9281-1

First, M. B., Williams, J. B., Karg, R. S., & Spitzer, R. L. (2016). *User's guide for the SCID-5-CV Structured Clinical Interview for DSM-5 disorders: Clinical version*. American Psychiatric Publishing.

Fischer, A. G., Bau, C. H., Grevet, E. H., Salgado, C. A., Victor, M. M., Kalil, K. L., Sousa, N. O., Garcia, C. R., & Belmonte-de-Abreu, P. (2007). The role of comorbid major depressive disorder in the clinical presentation of adult ADHD. *Journal of Psychiatric Research, 41*(12), 991–996. https://doi.org/10.1016/j.jpsychires.2006.09.008

Fossati, A., Novella, L., Donati, D., Donini, M., & Maffei, C. (2002). History of childhood attention deficit/hyperactivity disorder symptoms and borderline personality disorder: A controlled study. *Comprehensive Psychiatry, 43*(5), 369–377. https://doi.org/10.1053/comp.2002.34634

Franke, B., Faraone, S. V., Asherson, P., Buitelaar, J., Bau, C. H. D., Ramos-Quiroga, J. A., Mick, E., Grevet, E. H., Johansson, S., Haavik, J., Lesch, K. P., Cormand, B., Reif, A., & International Multicentre persistent ADHD CollaboraTion (IMpACT). (2012). The genetics of attention deficit/hyperactivity disorder in adults, a review. *Molecular Psychiatry, 17*(10), 960–987. https://doi.org/10.1038/mp.2011.138

Franz, A. P., Bolat, G. U., Bolat, H., Matijasevich, A., Santos, I. S., Silveira, R. C., Procianoy, R. S., Rohde, L. A., & Moreira-Maia, C. R. (2018). Attention-deficit/hyperactivity disorder and very preterm/very low birth weight: A meta-analysis. *Pediatrics, 141*(1), e20171645. https://doi.org/10.1542/peds.2017-1645

Fristad, M. A., Ackerman, J. P., & Nick, E. A. (2018). Adaptation of multi-family psychoeducational psychotherapy (MF-PEP) for adolescents with mood disorders: Preliminary findings. *Evidence-Based Practice in Child and Adolescent Mental Health, 3*(4), 252–262. https://doi.org/10.1080/23794925.2018.1509031

Fristad, M. A., & Roley-Roberts, M. E. (2021). Bipolar disorder. In R. J. Prinstein, E. A. Youngstrom, E. J. Mash, & R. A. Barkley (Eds.), *Treatment of disorders in childhood and adolescence* (pp. 212–257). Guilford Press.

Froehlich, T. E., Anixt, J. S., Loe, I. M., Chirdkiatgumchai, V., Kuan, L., & Gilman, R. C. (2011). Update on environmental risk factors for attention-deficit/hyperactivity disorder. *Current Psychiatry Reports, 13*(5), 333–344. https://doi.org/10.1007/s11920-011-0221-3

Geffen, J., & Forster, K. (2018). Treatment of ADHD in adults. *Therapeutic Advances in Vaccines and Immunotherapy, 8*, 25–32. https://doi.org/10.1177/2045125317734977

Gehricke, J. G., Kruggel, F., Thampipop, T., Alejo, S. D., Tatos, E., Fallon, J., & Muftuler, L. T. (2017). The brain anatomy of attention-deficit/hyperactivity disorder in young adults – a magnetic resonance imaging study. *PloS One, 12*(4), Article e0175433. https://doi.org/10.1371/journal.pone.0175433

Ginsberg, Y., Quintero, J., Anand, E., Casillas, M., & Upadhyaya, H. P. (2014). Underdiagnosis of attention-deficit/hyperactivity disorder in adult patients: A review of the literature. *Primary Care Companion for CNS Disorders, 16*(3), 23591. https://doi.org/10.4088/pcc.13r01600

Golden, C. J. (1978). *Stroop Color and Word Test: A manual for clinical and experimental uses.* Stoelting Company.

Graef, D. M., & Byars, K. C. (2021). Sleep problems. In M. J. Prinstein, E. A. Youngstrom, E. J. Mash, & R. A. Barkley (Eds.), *Treatment of disorders in childhood and adolesence* (pp. 807–862, 4th ed.). The Guilford Press.

Greenberg, L. M., & Waldman, I. D. (1993). Developmental normative data on the Test of Variables of Attention (T.O.V.A.). *Journal of Child Psychology and Psychiatry, and Allied Disciplines, 34*(6), 1019–1030. https://doi.org/10.1111/j.1469-7610.1993.tb01105.x

Groß-Lesch, S., Dempfle, A., Reichert, S., Jans, T., Geissler, J., Kittel-Schneider, S., Nguyen, T. T., Reif, A., Lesch, K. P., & Jacob, C. P. (2016). Sex- and subtype-related differences in the comorbidity of adult ADHDs. *Journal of Attention Disorders, 20*(10), 855–866. https://doi.org/10.1177/1087054713510353

Guo, N., Fuermaier, A. B. M., Koerts, J., Mueller, B. W., Diers, K., Mroß, A., Mette, C., Tucha, L., & Tucha, O. (2021). Neuropsychological functioning of individuals at clinical evaluation of adult ADHD. *Journal of Neural Transmission, 128*(7), 877–891. https://doi.org/10.1007/s00702-020-02281-0

Halperin, J. M., & Schulz, K. P. (2006). Revisiting the role of the prefrontal cortex in the pathophysiology of attention-deficit/hyperactivity disorder. *Psychological Bulletin, 132*(4), 560–581. https://doi.org/10.1037/0033-2909.132.4.560

Haltigan, J. D., & Vaillancourt, T. (2016). Identifying trajectories or borderline personality features in adolescence. *Canadian Journal of Psychiatry, 61*(3), 166–175. https://doi.org/10.1177/0706743715625953

Harpin, V., Mazzone, L., Raynaud, J. P., Kahle, J., & Hodgkins, P. (2016). Long-term outcomes of ADHD: A systematic review of self-esteem and social function. *Journal of Attention Disorders, 20*(4), 295–305. https://doi.org/10.1177/1087054713486516

Hinshaw, S. P., Owens, E. B., Zalecki, C., Huggins, S. P., Montenegro-Nevado, A. J., Schrodek, E., & Swanson, E. N. (2012). Prospective follow-up of girls with attention-deficit/hyperactivity disorder into early adulthood: Continuing impairment includes elevated risk for suicide attempts and self-injury. *Journal of Consulting and Clinical Psychology, 80*(6), 1041–1051. https://doi.org/10.1037/a0029451

Holst, Y., & Thorell, L. B. (2016). Neuropsychological functioning in adults with ADHD and adults with other psychiatric disorders: The issue of specificity. *Journal of Attention Disorders, 21*(2), 137–148. https://doi.org/10.1177/1087054713506264

Holst, Y., & Thorell, L. B. (2019). Functional impairments among adults with ADHD: A comparison with adults with other psychiatric disorders and links to executive deficits. *Applied Neuropsychology: Adult, 27*(3), 243–255. https://doi.org/10.1080/23279095.2018.1532429

Holthe, M. E. G., & Langvik, E. (2017). The strives, struggles, and successes of women diagnosed with ADHD as adults. *Sage Open, 7*(1), 2158244017701799. https://doi.org/10.1177/2158244017701799

Hong, M., Kooij, J. J. S., Kim, B., Joung, Y. S., Yoo, H. K., Kim, E. J., Lee, S. I., Bhang, S. Y., Lee, S. Y., Han, D. H., Lee, Y. S., & Bahn, G. H. (2020). Validity of the Korean version of DIVA-5: A semi-structured diagnostic interview for adult ADHD. *Neuropsychiatric Disease and Treatment, 16*, 2371-2376. https://doi.org/10.2147/ndt.s262995

Huang, A., Wu, K., Cai, Z., Lin, Y., Zhang, X., & Huang, Y. (2021). Association between postnatal second-hand smoke exposure and ADHD in children: A systematic review and meta-analysis. *Environmental Science Pollution Research International, 28*(2), 1370-1380. https://doi.org/10.1007/s11356-020-11269-y

Huang, H., Huang, H., Spottswood, M., & Ghaemi, N. (2020). Approach to evaluating and managing adult attention-deficit/hyperactivity disorder in primary care. *Harvard Review of Psychiatry, 28*(2), 100-106. https://doi.org/10.1097/hrp.0000000000000248

Humphreys, K. L., Eng, T., & Lee, S. S. (2013). Stimulant medication and substance use outcomes: A meta-analysis. *JAMA Psychiatry, 70*(7), 740-749. https://doi.org/10.1001/jamapsychiatry.2013.1273

Jensen, P. S., Hinshaw, S. P., Swanson, J. M., Greenhill, L. L., Conners, C. K., Arnold, L. E., Abikoff, H. B., Elliott, G., Hechtman, L., Hoza, B., March, J. S., Newcorn, J. H., Severe, J. B., Vitiello, B., Wells, K., & Wigal, T. (2001). Findings from the NIMH multimodal treatment study of ADHD (MTA): Implications and applications for primary care providers. *Journal of Developmental and Behavioral Pediatrics, 22*(1), 60-73. https://doi.org/10.1097/00004703-200102000-00008

Joshi, G., Petty, C., Wozniak, J., Faraone, S. V., Spencer, A. E., Woodworth, K. Y., Shelley-Abrahamson, R., McKillop, H., Furtak, S. L., & Biederman, J. (2013). A prospective open-label trial of paliperidone monotherapy for the treatment of bipolar spectrum disorders in children and adolescents. *Psychopharmacology, 227*(3), 449-458. https://doi.org/10.1007/s00213-013-2970-

Kapalka, G., Brown, R. T., Custis, D., Wu, T. C., & Marquez, M. (2018). Childhood and adolescent disorders: Evidence-based integrated biopsychosocial treatment of ADHD and disruptive disorders. In M. Muse (Ed.), *Cognitive behavioral psychopharmacology: The clinical practice of evidence-based biopsychosocial integration* (pp. 243-284). Wiley-Blackwell.

Kaplow, J. B., Layne, C. M., & Pynoos, R. S. (2021). Persistent complex bereavement disorder. In R. J. Prinstein, E. A. Youngstrom, E. J. Mash, & R. A. Barkley (Eds.), *Treatment of disorders in childhood and adolescence* (pp. 560-590). Guilford Press.

Katzman, M. A., Bilkey, T. S., Chokka, P. R., Fallu, A., & Klassen, L. J. (2017). Adult ADHD and comorbid disorders: Clinical implications of a dimensional approach. *BMC Psychiatry, 17*(1), 1-15. https://doi.org/10.1186/s12888-017-1463-3

Kessler, R. C., Adler, L., Ames, M., Demler, O., Faraone, S., Hiripi, E., Howes, M. J., Jin, R., Secnik, K., Spencer, T., Ustun, T. B., & Walters, E. E. (2005). The World Health Organization Adult ADHD Self-Report Scale (ASRS): A short screening scale for use in the general population. *Psychological Medicine, 35*(2), 245-256. https://doi.org/10.1017/s0033291704002892

Kessler, R. C., Adler, L., Barkley, R., Biederman, J., Conners, C. K., Demler, O., Faraone, S. V., Greenhill, L. L., Howes, M. J., Secnik, K., Spencer, T., Ustun, T. B., Walters, E. E., & Zaslavsky, A. M. (2006). The prevalence and correlates of adult ADHD in the United States: Results from the National Comorbidity Survey Replication. *American Journal of Psychiatry, 163*(4), 716-723. https://doi.org/10.1176/ajp.2006.163.4.716

Kessler, R. C., Adler, L. A., Gruber, M. J., Sarawate, C. A., Spencer, T., & Van Brunt, D. L. (2007). Validity of the World Health Organization Adult ADHD Self-Report Scale (ASRS) screener in a representative sample of health plan members. *International Journal of Methods in Psychiatric Research, 16*(2), 52-65. https://doi.org/10.1002/mpr.208

Kessler, R. C., Green, J. G., Adler, L. A., Barkley, R. A., Chatterji, S., Faraone, S. V., Finkelman, M., Greenhill, L. L., Gruber, M. J., Jewell, M., Russo, L. J., Sampson, N. A., & Van Brunt, D. L. (2010). Structure and diagnosis of adult attention-deficit/hyperactivity disorder: Analysis of expanded symptom criteria from the Adult ADHD Clinical Diagnostic Scale. *Archives of General Psychiatry, 67*(11), 1168-1178. https://doi.org/10.1001/archgenpsychiatry.2010.146

Kim, J. H., Kim, J. Y., Lee, J., Jeong, G. H., Lee, E., Lee, S., Lee, K. H., Kronbichler, A., Stubbs, B., Solmi, M., Koyanagi, A., Hong, S. H., Dragioti, E., Jacob, L., Brunoni, A. R., Carvalho, A. F., Radua, J., Thompson, T., Smith, L., ... Fusar-Poli, P. (2020). Environmental risk factors, protective factors, and peripheral biomarkers for ADHD: An umbrella review. *Lancet Psychiatry, 7*(11), 955-970. https://doi.org/10.1016/S2215-0366(20)30312-6

Knopik, V. S., Sparrow, E. P., Madden, P. A., Bucholz, K. K., Hudziak, J. J., Reich, W., Slutske, W. S., Grant, J. D., McLaughlin, T. L., Todorov, A., Todd, R. D., & Heath, A. C. (2005). Contributions of parental alcoholism, prenatal substance exposure, and genetic transmission to child ADHD risk: A female twin study. *Psychological Medicine, 35*(5), 625-635. https://doi.org/10.1017/s0033291704004155

Knouse, L. E. (2015). Cognitive-behavioral therapy for ADHD in college: Recommendations "hot off the press." *ADHD Report, 23*(5), 8-15. https://doi.org/10.1521/adhd.2015.23.5.8

Kolar, D., Keller, A., Golfinopoulos, M., Cumyn, L., Syer, C., & Hechtman, L. (2008). Treatment of adults with attention-deficit/hyperactivity disorder. *Neuropsychiatric Disease and Treatment, 4*(2), 389-403. https://doi.org/10.2147/ndt.s6985

Kooij, J. J. S., Bejerot, S., Blackwell, A., Caci, H., Casas-Brugué, M., Carpentier, P. J., Edvinsson, D., Fayyad, J., Foeken, K., Fitzgerald, M., Gaillac, V., Ginsberg, Y., Henry, C., Krause, J., Lensing, M. B., Manor, I., Niederhofer, H., Nunes-Filipe, C., Ohlmeier, M. D., ... Asherson, P. (2010). European consensus statement on diagnosis and treatment of adult ADHD: The European Network Adult ADHD. *BMC Psychiatry, 10*(1), 67-91. https://doi.org/10.1186/1471-244X-10-67

Kooij, J. J. S., Bijlenga, D., Salerno, L., Jaeschke, R., Bitter, I., Balázs, J., Thome, J., Dom, G., Kasper, S., Nunes Filipe, C., Stes, S., Mohr, P., Leppämäki, S., Casas, M., Bobes, J., McCarthy, J. M., Richarte, V., Kjems Philipsen, A., Pehlivanidis, A., ... Asherson, P. (2019). Updated European consensus statement on diagnosis and treatment of adult ADHD. *European Psychiatry, 56*(1), 14-34. https://doi.org/10.1016/j.eurpsy.2018.11.001

Kooij, J. J. S., & Francken, M. H. (2010). *DIVA 2.0: Diagnostic interview voor ADHD in adults bij volwassenen* [DIVA 2.0: Diagnostic Interview ADHD in Adults]. DIVA Foundation.

Korkman, M., Kirk, U., & Kemp, S. (2007). *NEPSY – Second edition (NEPSY-II)*. Harcourt Assessment.

La Malfa, G., Lassi, S., Bertelli, M., Pallanti, S., & Albertini, G. (2008). Detecting attention-deficit/hyperactivity disorder (ADHD) in adults with intellectual disability: The use of Conners' Adult ADHD Rating Scales (CAARS). *Research in Developmental Disabilities, 29*(2), 158-164. https://doi.org/10.1016/j.ridd.2007.02.002

Langberg, J. M., Epstein, J. N., & Graham, A. J. (2008). Organizational-skills interventions in the treatment of ADHD. *Expert Review of Neurotherapeutics, 8*(10), 1549-1561. https://doi.org/10.1586/14737175.8.10.1549

Larson, K., Russ, S. A., Kahn, R. S., & Halfon, N. (2011). *Patterns of comorbidity, functioning, and service use for US children with ADHD*, 2007. *Pediatrics, 127*(3), 462-470. https://doi.org/10.1542/peds.2010-0165

Lebowitz, M. S. (2013). Stigmatization of ADHD: A developmental review. *Journal of Attention Disorders, 20*(3), 199-205. https://doi.org/10.1177/1087054712475211

Lecrubier, Y., Sheehan, D., Weiller, E., Amorim, P., Bonora, I., Sheehan, K., Janavs, J., & Dunbar, G. (1997). The Mini International Neuropsychiatric Interview (MINI). A short diagnostic structured interview: Reliability and validity according to the

CIDI. *European Psychiatry, 12*(5), 224–231. https://doi.org/10.1016/S0924-9338(97)83296-8

León-Barriera, R., Ortegon, R. S., Chaplin, M. M., & Modesto-Lowe, V. (2022). Treating ADHD and comorbid anxiety in children: A guide for clinical practice. *Clinical Pediatrics, 62*(1), 39–46. https://doi.org/10.1177/00099228221111246

Li, T., Mota, N. R., Galesloot, T. E., Bralten, J., Buitelaar, J. K., IntHout, J., AriasVasquez, A., & Franke, B. (2019). ADHD symptoms in the adult general population are associated with factors linked to ADHD in adult patients. *European Neuropsychopharmacology, 29*(10), 1117–1126. https://doi.org/10.1016/j.euroneuro.2019.07.136

López-Pinar, C., Martínez-Sanchís, S., Carbonell-Vayá, E., Fenollar-Cortés, J., & Sánchez-Meca, J. (2018). Long-term efficacy of psychosocial treatments for adults with attention-deficit/hyperactivity disorder: A meta-analytic review. *Frontiers in Psychology, 9,* 638. https://doi.org/10.3389/fpsyg.2018.00638

Lotzin, A., Grundmann, J., Hiller, P., Pawils, S., & Schäfer, I. (2019). Profiles of childhood trauma in women with substance use disorders and comorbid posttraumatic stress disorders. *Frontiers in Psychiatry, 10,* Article 674. https://doi.org/10.3389/fpsyt.2019.00674

Lovett, B. J., & Harrison, A. G. (2021). Assessing adult ADHD: New research and perspectives. *Journal of Clinical and Experimental Neuropsychology, 43*(4), 333–339. https://doi.org/10.1080/13803395.2021.1950640

Manzari, N., Matvienko-Sikar, K., Baldoni, F., O'Keeffe, G. W., & Khashan, A. S. (2019). Prenatal maternal stress and risk of neurodevelopmental disorders in the offspring: A systematic review and meta-analysis. *Social Psychiatry and Psychiatric Epidemiology, 54*(11), 1299–1309. https://doi.org/10.1007/s00127-019-01745-3

Mapou, R. L. (2019). Counterpoint: Neuropsychological testing is not useful in the diagnosis of ADHD, but …. *ADHD Report, 27*(2), 8–12. https://doi.org/10.1521/adhd.2019.27.2.8

Marshall, P., Hoelzle, J., & Nikolas, M. (2021). Diagnosing attention-deficit/hyperactivity disorder (ADHD) in young adults: A qualitative review of the utility of assessment measures and recommendations for improving the diagnostic process. *Clinical Neuropsychologist, 35*(1), 165–198. https://doi.org/10.1080/13854046.2019.1696409

Mattingly, G. W., Wilson, J., Ugarte, L., & Glaser, P. (2021). Individualization of attention-deficit/hyperactivity disorder treatment: Pharmacotherapy considerations by age and co-occurring conditions. *CNS Spectrums, 26*(3), 202–221. https://doi.org/10.1017/s1092852919001822

McIntyre, R. S., Kennedy, S. H., Soczynska, J. K., Nguyen, H. T., Bilkey, T. S., Woldeyohannes, H. O., Nathanson, J. A., Joshi, S., Cheng, J. S., Benson, K. M., & Muzina, D. J. (2010). Attention-deficit/hyperactivity disorder in adults with bipolar disorder or major depressive disorder: Results from the international mood disorders collaborative project. *Primary Care Companion – Journal of Clinical Psychiatry, 12*(3), e1–e7. https://doi.org/10.4088/PCC.09m00861gry

McCann, B. S., Scheele, L., Ward, N., & Roy-Byrne, P. (2000). Discriminant validity of the Wender Utah Rating Scale for attention-deficit/hyperactivity disorder in adults. *Journal of Neuropsychiatry and Clinical Neurosciences, 12*(2), 240–245. https://doi.org/10.1176/jnp.12.2.240

McGough, J. J. (2016). Treatment controversies in adult ADHD. *American Journal of Psychiatry, 173*(10), 960–966. https://doi.org/10.1176/appi.ajp.2016.15091207

The MTA Cooperative Group. (1999). A 14-month randomized clinical trial of treatment strategies for attention-deficit/hyperactivity disorder. *Archives of General Psychiatry, 56*(12), 1073–1086. https://doi.org/10.1001/archpsyc.56.12.1073

Nierenberg, A. A., Miyahara, S., Spencer, T., Wisniewski, S. R., Otto, M. W., Simon, N., Pollack, M. H., Ostacher, M. J., Yan, L., Siegel, R., Sachs, G. S., & STEP-BD Investigators. (2005). Clinical and diagnostic implications of lifetime attention-deficit/hyperactivity disorder comorbidity in adults with bipolar disorder: Data from the first 1000 STEP-BD participants. *Biological Psychiatry, 57*(11), 1467–1473. https://doi.org/10.1016/j.biopsych.2005.01.036

Nigg, J. T. (2000). On inhibition/disinhibition in developmental psychopathology: Views from cognitive and personality psychology and a working inhibition taxonomy. *Psychological Bulletin, 126*(2), 220–246. https://doi.org/10.1037/0033-2909.126.2.220

Nigg, J. T., & Barkley, R. A. (2014). Attention-deficit/hyperactivity disorder. In E. J. Mash & R. A. Barkley (Eds.), *Child psychopathology* (3rd ed., pp. 75–144). Guilford Press.

Nikolas, M. A., Marshall, P., & Hoelzle, J. B. (2019). The role of neurocognitive tests in the assessment of adult attention-deficit/hyperactivity disorder. *Psychological Assessment, 31*(5), 685–698. https://doi.org/10.1037/pas0000688

Nordgaard, J., Sass, L. A., & Parnas, J. (2012). The psychiatric interview: Validity, structure, and subjectivity. *European Archives of Psychiatry and Clinical Neuroscience, 263*(4), 353–364. https://doi.org/10.1007/s00406-012-0366-z

O'Callaghan, P. (2014). Adherence to stimulants in adult ADHD. *ADHD Attention Deficit and Hyperactivity Disorders, 6*(2), 111–120. https://doi.org/10.1007/s12402-014-0129-y

Oosterloo, M., Lammers, G. J., Overeem, S., de Noord, I., & Kooij, J. J. (2006). Possible confusion between primary hypersomnia and adult attention-deficit/hyperactivity disorder. *Psychiatry Research, 143*(2-3), 293–297. https://doi.org/10.1016/j.psychres.2006.02.009

Osterrieth, P. A. (1944). Le test de copie d'une figure complexe: Contribution à l'étude de la perception et de la mémoire [Test of copying a complex figure: Contribution to the study of perception and memory]. *Archives de Psychologie, 30*, 206–356.

Owens, E., Cardoos, S. L., & Hinshaw, S. P. (2015). Developmental progression and gender differences among individuals with ADHD. In R. A. Barkley (Ed.), *Attention-deficit hyperactivity disorder: A handbook for diagnosis and treatment* (4th ed., pp. 223–255). Guilford Press.

Owens, J. A. (2008). Sleep disorders and attention-deficit/hyperactivity disorder. *Current Psychiatry Reports, 10*(5), 439–444. https://doi.org/10.1007/s11920-008-0070-x

Pedersen, E. M. J., Köhler-Forsberg, O., Nordentoft, M., Christensen, R. H. B., Mortensen, P. B., Petersen, L., & Benros, M. E. (2020). Infections of the central nervous system as a risk factor for mental disorders and cognitive impairment: A nationwide register-based study. *Brain, Behavior, and Immunity, 88*, 668–674. https://doi.org/https://doi.org/10.1016/j.bbi.2020.04.072

Pelham, W. E., Burrows-MacLean, L., Gnagy, E. M., Fabiano, G. A., Coles, E. K., Wymbs, B. T., Chacko, A., Walker, K. S., Wymbs, F., Garefino, A., Hoffman, M. T., Waxmonsky, J. G., & Waschbusch, D. A. (2014). A dose-ranging study of behavioral and pharmacological treatment in social settings for children with ADHD. *Journal of Abnormal Child Psychology, 42*(6), 1019–1031. https://doi.org/10.1007/s10802-013-9843-8

Perepletchikova, F., & Nathanson, D. (2021). Personality disorders. In R. J. Prinstein, E. A. Youngstrom, E. J. Mash, & R. A. Barkley (Eds.), *Treatment of disorders in childhood and adolescence* (pp. 560–590). Guilford Press.

Pievsky, M. A., & McGrath, R. E. (2018). The neurocognitive profile of attention-deficit/hyperactivity disorder: A review of meta-analyses. *Archives of Clinical Neuropsychology, 33*(2), 143–157. https://doi.org/10.1093/arclin/acx055

Piper, B. J., Ogden, C. L., Simoyan, O. M., Chung, D. Y., Caggiano, J. F., Nichols, S. D., & McCall, K. L. (2018). Trends in use of prescription stimulants in the United States and Territories, 2006 to 2016. *PloS One, 13*(11), e0206100. https://doi.org/10.1371/journal.pone.0206100

Power, T. J., Mautone, J. A., Soffer, S. L., Clarke, A. T., Marshall, S. A., Sharman, J., Blum, N. J., Glanzman, M., Elia, J., & Jawad, A. F. (2012). A family-school intervention for children with ADHD: Results of a randomized clinical trial. *Journal of*

*Consulting and Clinical Psychology, 80*(4), 611–623. https://doi.org/10.1037/a0028188

Pyman, P., Collins, S. E., Muggli, E., Testa, R., & Anderson, P. J. (2021). Cognitive and behavioural attention in children with low-moderate and heavy doses of prenatal alcohol exposure: A systematic review and meta-analysis. *Neuropsychology Review, 31*(4), 610–627. https://doi.org/10.1007/s11065-021-09490-8

Ramachandran, S., Dertien, D., & Bentley, S. I. (2020). Prevalence of ADHD symptom malingering, nonmedical use, and drug diversion among college-enrolled adults with a prescription for stimulant medications. *Journal of Addictive Diseases, 38*(2), 176–185. https://doi.org/10.1080/10550887.2020.1732762

Ramos-Quiroga, J. A., Nasillo, V., Richarte, V., Corrales, M., Palma, F., Ibáñez, P., Michelsen, M., Van de Glind, G., Casas, M., & Kooij, J. J. S. (2019). Criteria and concurrent validity of DIVA 2.0: A semi-structured diagnostic interview for adult ADHD. *Journal of Attention Disorders, 23*(10), 1126–1135. https://doi.org/10.1177/1087054716646451

Rieppi, R., Greenhill, L. L., Ford, R. E., Chuang, S., Wu, M., Davies, M., Abikoff, H. B., Arnold, L. E., Conners, C. K., Elliott, G. R., Hechtman, L., Hinshaw, S. P., Hoza, B., Jensen, P. S., Kraemer, H. C., March, J. S., Newcorn, J. H., Pelham, W. E., Severe, J. B., ... Wigal, T. (2002). Socioeconomic status as a moderator of ADHD treatment outcomes. *Journal of the American Academy of Child & Adolescent Psychiatry, 41*(3), 269–277. https://doi.org/10.1097/00004583-200203000-00006

Roberts, R. E., Roberts, C. R., & Xing, Y. (2007). Comorbidity of substance use disorders and other psychiatric disorders among adolescents: Evidence from an epidemiologic survey. *Drug and Alcohol Dependence, 88*(Suppl. 1), S4–S13. https://doi.org/10.1016/j.drugalcdep.2006.12.010

Rostain, A. L., Diaz, Y., & Pedraza, J. (2015). Solutions for treating Hispanic adults with ADHD. *Journal of Clinical Psychiatry, 76*(2), 19848. https://doi.org/10.4088/jcp.13009co6c

Rostain, A. L., & Ramsay, J. R. (2006). A combined treatment approach for adults with ADHD – results of an open study of 43 patients. *Journal of Attention Disorders, 10*(2), 150–159. https://doi.org/10.1177/1087054706288110

Rostain, A. L., Ramsay, J. R., & Waite, R. (2015). Culturally competent strategies for assessing and treating ADHD in African American adults. *Journal of Clinical Psychiatry, 76*(5), 592–596. https://doi.org/10.4088/jcp.13008co6c

Rubia K. (2018). Cognitive neuroscience of attention deficit hyperactivity disorder (ADHD) and its clinical translation. *Frontiers in Human Neuroscience, 12*, Article 100. https://doi.org/10.3389/fnhum.2018.00100

Rutter, M., Cox, A., Tupling, C., Berger, M., & Yule, W. (1975). Attainment and adjustment in two geographical areas. I. The prevalence of psychiatric disorder. *British Journal of Psychiatry, 126*(6), 493–509. https://doi.org/10.1192/bjp.126.6.493

Safren, S. A., Otto, M. W., Sprich, S., Winett, C. L., Wilens, T. E., & Biederman, J. (2005). Cognitive-behavioral therapy for ADHD in medication-treated adults with continued symptoms. *Behaviour Research and Therapy, 43*(7), 831–842. https://doi.org/10.1016/j.brat.2004.07.001

Sagvolden, T., Johansen, E. B., Aase, H., & Russell, V. A. (2005). A dynamic developmental theory of attention-deficit/hyperactivity disorder (ADHD) predominantly hyperactive/impulsive and combined subtypes. *Behavioral and Brain Sciences, 28*(3), 397–468. https://doi.org/10.1017/S0140525X05000075

Sahakian, B. J., Morris, R. G., Evenden, J. L., Heald, A., Levy, R., Philpot, M., & Robbins, T. W. (1988). A comparative study of visuospatial memory and learning in Alzheimer-type dementia and Parkinson's disease. *Brain: A Journal of Neurology, 111*(Pt. 3), 695–718. https://doi.org/10.1093/brain/111.3.695

San Martin Porter, M., Maravilla, J. C., Betts, K. S., & Alati, R. (2019). Low-moderate prenatal alcohol exposure and offspring attention-deficit hyperactivity disorder (ADHD): Systematic review and meta-analysis. *Archives of Gynecology and Obstetrics, 300*(2), 269–277. https://doi.org/10.1007/s00404-019-05204-x

Scheffer, R. E., Kowatch, R. A., Carmody, T., & Rush, A. J. (2005). Randomized placebo-controlled trial of mixed amphetamine salts for symptoms of comorbid ADHD in pediatric bipolar disorder after mood stabilization with divalproex sodium. *American Journal of Psychiatry, 162*(1), 58–64. https://doi.org/10.1176/appi.ajp.162.1.58

Schein, J., Childress, A., Adams, J., Cloutier, M., Gagnon-Sanschagrin, P., Maitland, J., Bungay, R., Guérin, A., & Lefebvre, P. (2021). Treatment patterns among adults with attention-deficit/hyperactivity disorder in the United States: A retrospective claims study. *Current Medical Research and Opinion, 37*(11), 2007–2014. https://doi.org/10.1080/03007995.2021.1968814

Schneider, M., Retz, W., Coogan, A., Thome, J., & Rösler, M. (2006). Anatomical and functional brain imaging in adult attention-deficit/hyperactivity disorder (ADHD): A neurological view. *European Archives of Psychiatry and Clinical Neuroscience, 256*(Suppl. 1), i32–i41. https://doi.org/10.1007/s00406-006-1005-3

Schoenfelder, E. N., Faraone, S. V., & Kollins, S. H. (2014). Stimulant treatment of ADHD and cigarette smoking: A meta-analysis. *Pediatrics, 133*(6), 1070–1080. https://doi.org/10.1542/peds.2014-0179

Sciberras, E., Mulraney, M., Silva, D., & Coghill, D. (2017). Prenatal risk factors and the etiology of ADHD: Review of existing evidence. *Current Psychiatry Reports, 19*(1), Article 1. https://doi.org/10.1007/s11920-017-0753-2

Sharma, M. J., Lavoie, S., & Callahan, B. L. (2021). A call for research on the validity of the age-of-onset criterion application in older adults being evaluated for ADHD: A review of the literature in clinical and cognitive psychology. *American Journal of Geriatric Psychiatry, 29*(7), 669–678. https://doi.org/10.1016/j.jagp.2020.10.016

Shaw, M., Hodgkins, P., Caci, H., Young, S., Kahle, J., Woods, A. G., & Arnold, L. E. (2012). A systematic review and analysis of long-term outcomes in attention deficit hyperactivity disorder: Effects of treatment and non-treatment. *BMC Medicine, 10*, Article 99. https://doi.org/10.1186/1741-7015-10-99

Shen, C., Luo, Q., Jia, T., Zhao, Q., Desrivières, S., Quinlan, E. B., Banaschewski, T., Millenet, S., Bokde, A. L. W., Büchel, C., Flor, H., Frouin, V., Garavan, H., Gowland, P., Heinz, A., Ittermann, B., Martinot, J. L., Artiges, E., Paillère-Martinot, M. L., ... IMAGEN consortium. (2020). Neural correlates of the dual-pathway model for ADHD in adolescents. *American Journal of Psychiatry, 177*(9), 844–854. https://doi.org/10.1176/appi.ajp.2020.19020183

Sibley, M. H. (2021). Empirically-informed guidelines for first-time adult ADHD diagnosis. *Journal of Clinical and Experimental Neuropsychology, 43*(4), 340–351. https://doi.org/10.1080/13803395.2021.1923665

Sibley, M. H., Arnold, L. E., Swanson, J. M., Hechtman, L. T., Kennedy, T. M., Owens, E., Molina, B. S. G., Jensen, P. S., Hinshaw, S. P., Roy, A., Chronis-Tuscano, A., Newcorn, J. H., Rohde, L. A., & MTA Cooperative Group. (2022). Variable patterns of remission from ADHD in the multimodal treatment study of ADHD. *American Journal of Psychiatry, 179*(2), 142–151. https://doi.org/10.1176/appi.ajp.2021.21010032

Sibley, M. H., Kuriyan, A. B., Evans, S. W., Waxmonsky, J. G., & Smith, B. H. (2014). Pharmacological and psychosocial treatments for adolescents with ADHD: An updated systematic review of the literature. *Clinical Psychology Review, 34*(3), 218–232. https://doi.org/10.1016/j.cpr.2014.02.001

Sibley, M. H., Mitchell, J. T., & Becker, S. P. (2016). Method of adult diagnosis influences estimated persistence of childhood ADHD: A systematic review of longitudinal studies. *Lancet Psychiatry, 3*(12), 1157–1165. https://doi.org/10.1016/s2215-0366(16)30190-0

Sibley, M. H., Rohde, L. A., Swanson, J. M., Hechtman, L. T., Molina, B. S. G., Mitchell, J. T., Arnold, L. E., Caye, A., Kennedy, T. M., Roy, A., Stehli, A., & Multimodal Treatment Study of Children with ADHD (MTA) Cooperative Group. (2018). Late-onset ADHD reconsidered with comprehensive repeated assessments between ages 10 and 25. *American Journal of Psychiatry, 175*(2), 140–149. https://doi.org/10.1176/appi.ajp.2017.17030298

Silva, D., & Ibilola, O. (2021). Environmental (perinatal) risk factors of ADHD in a sibling control design study. *Open Access Journal of Behavioural Science & Psychology, 4*(1), 180052.

Silverstein, M. J., Faraone, S. V., Alperin, S., Leon, T. L., Biederman, J., Spencer, T. J., & Adler, L. A. (2018). Validation of the expanded versions of the Adult ADHD Self-Report Scale v1.1 symptom checklist and the adult ADHD investigator symptom rating scale. *Journal of Attention Disorders, 23*(10), 1101–1110. https://doi.org/10.1177/1087054718756198

Silverstein, M. J., Faraone, S. V., Leon, T. L., Biederman, J., Spencer, T. J., & Adler, L. A. (2020). The relationship between executive function deficits and DSM-5-defined ADHD symptoms. *Journal of Attention Disorders, 24*(1), 41–51. https://doi.org/10.1177/1087054718804347

Simon, V., Czobor, P., Bálint, S., Mészáros, Á, & Bitter, I. (2009). Prevalence and correlates of adult attention-deficit hyperactivity disorder: Meta-analysis. *British Journal of Psychiatry, 194*(3), 204–211. https://doi.org/10.1192/bjp.bp.107.048827

Solanto, M. V., Marks, D. J., Mitchell, K. J., Wasserstein, J., & Kofman, M. D. (2008). Development of a new psychosocial treatment for adult ADHD. *Journal of Attention Disorders, 11*(6), 728–736. https://doi.org/10.1177/1087054707305100

Solanto, M. V., Marks, D. J., Wasserstein, J., Mitchell, K., Abikoff, H., Alvir, J. M., & Kofman, M. D. (2010). Efficacy of meta-cognitive therapy for adult ADHD. *American Journal of Psychiatry, 167*(8), 958–968. https://doi.org/10.1176/appi.ajp.2009.09081123

Stepp, S. D., Keenan, K., Hipwell, A. E., Krueger, R. F. (2014). The impact of childhood temperament on the development of borderline personality disorder symptoms over the course of adolescence. *Borderline Personality Disorder and Emotion Regulation, 1*, Article 18. https://doi.org/10.1186/2051-6673-1-18

Stevens, J. R., Wilens, T. E., & Stern, T. A. (2013). Using stimulants for attention-deficit/hyperactivity disorder: Clinical approaches and challenges. *Primary Care Companion for CNS Disorders, 15*(2). https://doi.org/10.4088/pcc.12f01472

Stroop, J. R. (1935). Studies of interference in serial verbal reactions. *Journal of Experimental Psychology, 18*(6), 643–662. https://doi.org/10.1037/h0054651

Subcommittee on Attention-Deficit/Hyperactivity Disorder, Steering Committee on Quality Improvement and Management. (2011). ADHD: Clinical practice guideline for the diagnosis, evaluation, and treatment of attention-deficit/hyperactivity disorder in children and adolescents. *Pediatrics, 128*(5), 1007–1022. https://doi.org/10.1542/peds.2011-2654

Surman, C. B. H. (2013). Clinical assessment of ADHD in adults. In C. B. H. Surman (Ed.), *ADHD in adults: A practical guide to evaluation and management* (pp. 19–44). Humana Press. https://doi.org/10.1007/978-1-62703-248-3_2

Surman, C. B. H., Hammerness, P. G., Pion, K., & Faraone, S. V. (2013). Do stimulants improve functioning in adults with ADHD? A review of the literature. *European Neuropsychopharmocology, 23*(6), 528–533. https://doi.org/10.1016/j.euroneuro.2012.02.010

Swanson, J. M., Kraemer, H. C., Hinshaw, S. P., Arnold, L. E., Conners, C. K., Abikoff, H. B., Clevenger, W., Davies, M., Elliott, G. R., Greenhill, L. L., Hechtman, L., Hoza, B., Jensen, P. S., March, J. S., Newcorn, J. H., Owens, E. B., Pelham, W. E., Schiller, E., Severe, J. B., ... Wu, M. (2001). Clinical relevance of the primary findings of the MTA: Success rates based on severity of ADHD and ODD symptoms at the end of treatment. *Journal of the American Academy of Child & Adolescent Psychiatry, 40*(2), 168–179. https://doi.org/10.1097/00004583-200102000-00011

Tamm, L., Denton, C. A., Epstein, J. N., Schatschneider, C., Taylor, H., Arnold, L. E., Bukstein, O., Anixt, J., Koshy, A., Newman, N. C., Maltinsky, J., Brinson, P., Loren, R. E. A., Prasad, M. R., Ewing-Cobbs, L., & Vaughn, A. (2017). Comparing treatments for children with ADHD and word reading difficulties: A randomized clinical trial. *Journal of Consulting and Clinical Psychology, 85*(5), 434–446. https://doi.org/10.1037/ccp0000170

Tannock, R., Frijters, J. C., Martinussen, R., White, E. J., Ickowicz, A., Benson, N. J., & Lovett, M. W. (2018). Combined modality intervention for ADHD with comorbid reading disorders: A proof of concept study. *Journal of Learning Disabilities, 51*(1), 55-72. https://doi.org/10.1177/0022219416678409

Targum, S. D., & Adler, L. A. (2014). Our current understanding of adult ADHD. *Innovations in Clinical Neuroscience, 11*(11-12), 30-35.

Taylor, E. (2011). Antecedents of ADHD: A historical account of diagnostic concepts. *ADHD Attention Deficit and Hyperactivity Disorders, 3*(2), 69-75. https://doi.org/10.1007/s12402-010-0051-x

Thapar, A., Cooper, M., Eyre, O., & Langley, K. (2013). What have we learnt about the causes of ADHD? *Journal of Child Psychology and Psychiatry, 54*(1), 3-16. https://doi.org/10.1111/j.1469-7610.2012.02611.x

Theiling, J., & Petermann, F. (2016). Neuropsychological profiles on the WAIS-IV of adults with ADHD. *Journal of Attention Disorders, 20*(11), 913-924. https://doi.org/10.1177/1087054713518241

Torgersen, T., Gjervan, B., & Rasmussen, K. (2006). ADHD in adults: A study of clinical characteristics, impairment and comorbidity. *Nordic Journal of Psychiatry, 60*(1), 38-43. https://doi.org/10.1080/08039480500520665

Torgersen, T., Gjervan, B., & Rasmussen, K. (2008). Treatment of adult ADHD: Is current knowledge useful to clinicians? *Neuropsychiatric Disease and Treatment, 4*(1), 177-186.

Tourjman, V., Louis-Nascan, G., Ahmed, G., DuBow, A., Côté, H., Daly, N., Daoud, G., Espinet, S., Flood, J., Gagnier-Marandola, E., Gignac, M., Graziosi, G., Mansuri, Z., & Sadek, J. (2022). Psychosocial interventions for attention deficit/hyperactivity disorder: A systematic review and meta-analysis by the CADDRA guidelines work group. *Brain Sciences, 12*(8), Article 1023. https://doi.org/10.3390/brainsci12081023

Trenerry, M., Crosson, B., Deboe, J., & Leber, W. (1989). *Stroop Neuropsychological Screening Test*. Psychological Assessment Resources.

Tripp, G., & Wickens, J. R. (2008). Research review: Dopamine transfer deficit: A neurobiological theory of altered reinforcement mechanisms in ADHD. *Journal of Child Psychology and Psychiatry, and Allied Disciplines, 49*(7), 691-704. https://doi.org/10.1111/j.1469-7610.2007.01851.x

Verbeeck, W., Bekkering, G. E., Van den Noortgate, W., & Kramers, C. (2017). Bupropion for attention deficit hyperactivity disorder (ADHD) in adults. *Cochrane Database of Systematic Reviews, 10*(10). https://doi.org/10.1002/14651858.CD009504.pub2

Vesco, A. T., Lehmann, J., Gracious, B. L., Arnold, L. E., & Fristad, M. A. (2015). Omega-3 supplementation for psychotic mania and comorbid anxiety in children: Review and case presentation. *Journal of Child and Adolescent Psychopharmacology, 25*(7), 526-534. https://doi.org/10.1089/cap.2013.0141

Vidal-Estrada, R., Bosch-Munso, R., Nogueira-Morais, M., Casas-Brugue, M., & Ramos-Quiroga, J. A. (2012). Psychological treatment of attention deficit hyperactivity disorder in adults: A systematic review. *Actas Espanolas de Psiquiatria, 40*(3), 147-154.

Vitola, E. S., Bau, C. H., Salum, G. A., Horta, B. L., Quevedo, L., Barros, F. C., Pinheiro, R. T., Kieling, C., Rohde, L. A., & Grevet, E. H. (2017). Exploring DSM-5 ADHD criteria beyond young adulthood: Phenomenology, psychometric properties and prevalence in a large three-decade birth cohort. *Psychological Medicine, 47*(4), 744-754. https://doi.org/10.1017/s0033291716002853

Volkow, N. D., Fowler, J. S., Wang, G., Ding, Y., & Gatley, S. J. (2002). Mechanism of action of methylphenidate: Insights from PET imaging studies. *Journal of Attention Disorders, 6*(Suppl. 1), S31-S43. https://doi.org/10.1177/070674370200601s05

Waite, R., & Ramsay, J. R. (2010). Adults with ADHD: Who are we missing? *Issues in Mental Health Nursing, 31*(10), 670-678. https://doi.org/10.3109/01612840.2010.496137

Wechsler, D. (2008). *Wechsler Adult Intelligence Scale - Fourth edition (WAIS-IV)*. NCS Pearson.

Wechsler, D. (2009). *Wechsler Memory Scale WMS-IV: Technical and interpretive manual*. Pearson.

Weiner, L., Perroud, N., & Weibel, S. (2019). Attention deficit hyperactivity disorder and borderline personality disorder in adults: A review of their links and risks. *Neuropsychiatric Disease and Treatment, 15*, 3115-3129. https://doi.org/10.2147/ndt.s192871

Weiss, M., Safren, S. A., Solanto, M. V., Hechtman, L., Rostain, A. L., Ramsay, J. R., & Murray, C. (2008). Research forum on psychological treatment of adults with ADHD. *Journal of Attention Disorders, 11*(6), 642-651. https://doi.org/10.1177/1087054708315063

Weyandt, L. L., & DuPaul, G. (2006). ADHD in college students. *Journal of Attention Disorders, 10*(1), 9-19. https://doi.org/10.1177/1087054705286061

Wilens, T. E., Biederman, J., Faraone, S. V., Martelon, M., Westerberg, D., & Spencer, T. J. (2009). Presenting ADHD symptoms, subtypes, and comorbid disorders in clinically referred adults with ADHD. *Journal of Clinical Psychiatry, 70*(11), 1557-1562. https://doi.org/10.4088/JCP.08m04785pur

Williamson, D., & Johnston, C. (2015). Gender differences in adults with attention-deficit/hyperactivity disorder: A narrative review. *Clinical Psychology Review, 40*, 15-27. https://doi.org/10.1016/j.cpr.2015.05.005

Wolfe, V. V., & Kelly, B. M. (2021). Child maltreatment. In R. J. Prinstein, E. A. Youngstrom, E. J. Mash, & R. A. Barkley (Eds.), *Treatment of disorders in childhood and adolescence* (pp. 592-657). Guilford Press.

World Health Organization. (2019). *International statistical classification of diseases and related health problems* (10th ed.). https://icd.who.int/browse10/2019/en#/F90-F98

World Health Organization. (2021). *International classification of diseases* (10th rev., clinical modification).

Yolton, K., Cornelius, M., Ornoy, A., McGough, J., Makris, S., & Schantz, S. (2014). Exposure to neurotoxicants and the development of attention deficit hyperactivity disorder and its related behaviors in childhood. *Neurotoxicology and Teratology, 44*, 30-45. https://doi.org/10.1016/j.ntt.2014.05.003

Yoshimasu, K., Barbaresi, W. J., Colligan, R. C., Voigt, R. G., Killian, J. M., Weaver, A. L., & Katusic, S. K. (2016). Adults with persistent ADHD: Gender and psychiatric comorbidities – a population-based longitudinal study. *Journal of Attention Disorders, 22*(6), 535-546. https://doi.org/10.1177/1087054716676342

# 8

# Appendix: Tools and Resources

The following materials for your book can be downloaded free of charge once you register on the Hogrefe website:

Appendix 1: Support Groups, Organizations, and Resources

DOWNLOAD

**How to proceed:**

1. Go to www.hgf.io/media and create a user account. If you already have one, please log in.

2. Go to **My supplementary materials** in your account dashboard and enter the code below. You will automatically be redirected to the download area, where you can access and download the supplementary materials.

   **Code: B-BPCGK6**

To make sure you have permanent direct access to all the materials, we recommend that you download them and save them on your computer.

# Appendix 1: Support Groups, Organizations, and Resources

This is a **preview** of the content that is available in the downloadable material of this book. Please see p. 89 for instructions on how to obtain the full-sized, printable PDF.

**One ADD Place**
Website: https://www.oneaddplace.com
Provides information for families of children and adults with. Offers information on both child and adult ADHD.

**ADD Warehouse**
3200 Northwest 70th Ave., Suite 102
Plantation, FL 33317
USA
Tel: +1 (800) 233-9273
Website: https://www.addwarehouse.com
A central location for ordering books, tapes, assessment scales, and videos selected to help parents, educators, and health professionals assist people affected by developmental disorders and ADHD.

**Center for Mental Health Services**
5600 Fishers Lane, Rm 15-105
Rockville, MD 20857
USA
Tel: +1 (800) 789-2647
Website: https://www.samhsa.gov/about-us/who-we-are/offices-centers/cmhs
A branch of the US Department of Health and Human Services that provides a range of information on mental health, treatment, and support services.

**Children and Adults with Attention Deficit Disorders (CHADD)**
8181 Professional Place, Suite 150
Landover, MD 20785
USA
Tel: +1 (800) 233-4050
Website: https://chadd.org/
This national nonprofit organization provides education, advocacy, and support for individuals with ADHD. In addition to CHADD's informative website, it also publishes a variety of printed materials, including *Attention* magazine, a free newsletter, and other publications on research advances and treatments for ADHD.

**National Institute of Mental Health**
6001 Executive Blvd.
Rockville, MD 20852
Tel: +1 (301) 443-4513 or +1 (866) 615-6464
Website: https://www.nimh.nih.gov/
A comprehensive resource for information based on research advances in brain, behavior, and mental illness. Provides information on ADHD assessment, diagnosis, treatment, and clinical trials.

**Dr. Hallowell: Live a Better Life**
https://drhallowell.com/

**Attention Deficit Disorder Association: Helping Adults With ADHD Lead Better Lives**
https://add.org/

**National Resource Center on ADHD: A Program of CHADD**
https://d393uh8gb46l22.cloudfront.net/wp-content/uploads/2021/12/NRC-Brochure-2021.pdf

**The American Professional Society of ADHD and Related Disorders (APSARD)**
https://apsard.org/

# Quick and comprehensive information on psychotropic drugs for adults

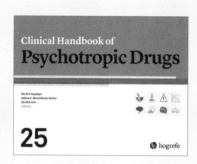

25th ed. 2023, iv + 484 pages + 38 printable PDF patient information sheets
$99.80 / € 84.95
ISBN 978-0-88937-632-8
Also available as eBook

*Also available as online version*

Ric M. Procyshyn / Kalyna Z. Bezchlibnyk-Butler / David D. Kim (Eds.)

## Clinical Handbook of Psychotropic Drugs

The *Clinical Handbook of Psychotropic Drugs* has become a standard reference and working tool for psychiatrists, psychologists, physicians, pharmacists, nurses, and other mental health professionals.

- Independent, unbiased, up-to-date
- Packed with unique, easy-to-read comparison charts and tables for a quick overview of treatment options
- Succinct, bulleted information on all classes of medication: on- and off-label indications, (US FDA, Health Canada), recommended dosages, US and Canadian trade names, side effects, interactions, pharmacodynamics, precautions in the young, the elderly, and pregnancy, nursing implications, and much more
- Potential interactions and side effects summarized in comparison charts
- With instantly recognizable icons and in full color throughout
- Clearly written patient information sheets available for download as printable PDF files

This book is a must for everyone who needs an up-to-date, easy-to-use, comprehensive summary of all the most relevant information about psychotropic drugs.

www.hogrefe.com

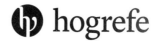

# Advances in Psychotherapy – Evidence-Based Practice

Developed and edited with the support of the Society of Clinical Psychology (APA Division 12)

**Editor-in-chief**
Danny Wedding, PhD, MPH

**Associate editors**
Jonathan S. Comer, PhD
Linda Carter Sobell, PhD, ABPP
Kenneth E. Freedland, PhD
J. Kim Penberthy, PhD, ABPP

- *Practice-oriented*
- *Evidence-based*
- *Expert authors*
- *Easy-to-read*
- *Compact*
- *Cost-effective*

*Latest releases*

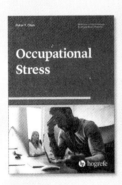

Occupational Stress

Volume 51

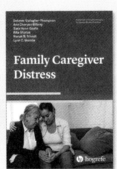

Family Caregiver Distress

Volume 50

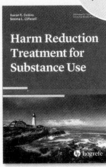

Harm Reduction Treatment for Substance Use

Volume 49

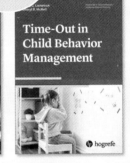

Time-Out in Child Behavior Management

Volume 48

www.hogrefe.com

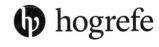

# Advances in Psychotherapy – Evidence-Based Practice

**All volumes of the series at a glance**

Affirmative Counseling for Transgender and Gender Diverse Clients (Vol. 45)
Alcohol Use Disorders (Vol. 10)
Alzheimer's Disease and Dementia (Vol. 38)
ADHD in Adults, 2nd ed., (Vol. 35)
ADHD in Children and Adolescents, 2nd. ed., (Vol. 33)
Autism Spectrum Disorder (Vol. 29)
Binge Drinking and Alcohol Misuse Among College Students and Young Adults (Vol. 32)
Bipolar Disorder (Vol. 1, 2nd ed.)
Body Dysmorphic Disorder (Vol. 44)
Childhood Maltreatment (Vol. 4, 2nd ed.)
Childhood Obesity (Vol. 39)
Chronic Illness in Children and Adolescents (Vol. 9)
Chronic Pain (Vol. 11)
Depression (Vol. 18)
Eating Disorders (Vol. 13)
Elimination Disorders in Children and Adolescents (Vol. 16)
Family Caregiver Distress (Vol. 50)
Generalized Anxiety Disorder (Vol. 24)
Growing Up with Domestic Violence (Vol. 23)
Harm Reduction Treatment for Substance Use (Vol. 49)
Headache (Vol. 30)
Heart Disease (Vol. 2)
Hoarding Disorder (Vol. 40)
Hypochondriasis and Health Anxiety (Vol. 19)
Insomnia (Vol. 42)
Integrating Digital Tools into Children's Mental Health Care (Vol. 52)
Internet Addiction (Vol. 41)
Language Disorders in Children and Adolescents (Vol. 28)
Mindfulness (Vol. 37)
Multiple Sclerosis (Vol. 36)
Nicotine and Tobacco Dependence (Vol. 21)
Nonsuicidal Self-Injury (Vol. 22)
Obsessive-Compulsive Disorder in Adults (Vol. 31)
Occupational Stress (Vol. 51)
Persistent Depressive Disorders (Vol. 43)
Phobic and Anxiety Disorders in Children and Adolescents (Vol. 27)
Problem and Pathological Gambling (Vol. 8)
Psychological Approaches to Cancer Care (Vol. 46)
Public Health Tools for Practicing Psychologists (Vol. 20)
Sexual Dysfunction in Women (Vol. 25)
Sexual Dysfunction in Men (Vol. 26)
Sexual Violence (Vol. 17)
Social Anxiety Disorder (Vol. 12)
Substance Use Problems (Vol. 15, 2nd ed.)
Suicidal Behavior (Vol. 14, 2nd ed.)
The Schizophrenia Spectrum (Vol. 5, 2nd ed.)
Time-Out in Child Behavior Management (Vol. 48)
Treating Victims of Mass Disaster and Terrorism (Vol. 6)
Women and Drinking: Preventing Alcohol-Exposed Pregnancies (Vol. 34)

**Prices:** US $29.80 / € 24.95 per volume. Standing order price US $24.80 / € 19.95 per volume (minimum 4 successive volumes) + postage & handling. Special rates for APA Division 12 and Division 42 members

www.hogrefe.com/apt

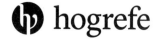

# How to assess and treat children and adolescents with ADHD effectively

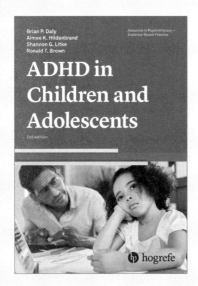

2024, viii + 92 pp.
$29.80 / € 24.95
ISBN 978-0-88937-600-7
Also available as eBook

Brian P. Daly / Aimee K. Hildenbrand / Shannon G. Litke / Ronald T. Brown

## ADHD in Children and Adolescents

This updated new edition of this popular text integrates the latest research and practices to give practitioners concise and readable guidance on the assessment and effective treatment of children and adolescents with attention-deficit/hyperactivity disorder (ADHD). This common childhood condition can have serious consequences for academic, emotional, social, and occupational functioning. When properly identified and diagnosed, however, there are many interventions that have established benefits.

This volume is both a compact "how to" reference, for use by professionals in their daily work, and an ideal educational reference for students. It has a similar structure to other books in the Advances in Psychotherapy series, and informs the reader of all aspects involved in the assessment and management of ADHD. Practitioners will particularly appreciate new information on the best approaches to the ideal sequencing of treatments in multimodal care, and the important diversity considerations. Suggestions for further reading, support groups, and educational organizations are also provided.

www.hogrefe.com

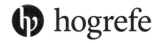